ROUTLEDGE LIBRARY EDITIONS: HEALTH, DISEASE & SOCIETY

Volume

PHARMACEUTICALS AND HEALTH POLICY

PHARMACEUTICALS AND HEALTH POLICY

International Perspectives on Provision and Control of Medicines

Editors
RICHARD BLUM,
ANDREW HERXHEIMER,
CATHERINE STENZL and
JASPER WOODCOCK

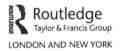
Routledge
Taylor & Francis Group

LONDON AND NEW YORK

First published in 1981 by Croom Helm Ltd.

This edition first published in 2022
by Routledge
4 Park Square, Milton Park, Abingdon, Oxon OX14 4RN

and by Routledge
605 Third Avenue, New York, NY 10158

Routledge is an imprint of the Taylor & Francis Group, an informa business

British Library Cataloguing in Publication Data
A catalogue record for this book is available from the British Library

ISBN: 978-0-367-52469-2 (Set)
ISBN: 978-1-032-25212-4 (Volume 5) (hbk)
ISBN: 978-1-032-25221-6 (Volume 5) (pbk)
ISBN: 978-1-003-28214-3 (Volume 5) (ebk)

DOI: 10.4324/9781003282143

Publisher's Note
The publisher has gone to great lengths to ensure the quality of this reprint but points out that some imperfections in the original copies may be apparent.

Disclaimer
The publisher has made every effort to trace copyright holders and would welcome correspondence from those they have been unable to trace.

PHARMACEUTICALS AND HEALTH POLICY

INTERNATIONAL PERSPECTIVES ON PROVISION AND CONTROL OF MEDICINES

EDITORS: RICHARD BLUM, ANDREW HERXHEIMER, CATHERINE STENZL, JASPER WOODCOCK

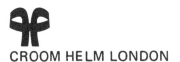

CROOM HELM LONDON

INTERNATIONAL RESEARCH GROUP FOR DRUG LEGISLATION AND PROGRAMS

© 1981 International Research Group for Drug Legislation and Programs
Croom Helm Ltd, 2-10 St John's Road, London SW11

British Library Cataloguing in Publication Data
Pharmaceuticals and health policy.
    1. Pharmaceutical policy
    I. Blum, Richard
    II. International Research Group for Drug
    Legislation and Programs
    362.1   RA401

To Lynn Pan who kept us all on course

Typeset by Leaper and Gard Ltd, Bristol
Printed and bound in Great Britain
by Billing and Sons Limited
Guildford, London, Oxford, Worcester

CONTENTS

NOTES ON CONTRIBUTORS

Anil Agarwal Assistant Director, Earthscan, London.

Michael E. Allan Director of Development, TIL (Medical), Ltd. London.

Carol Barker Lecturer in Health Services Planning, Nuffield Centre for Health Services Studies, University of Leeds. Formerly: Cabinet of Studies, Ministry of Health, Mozambique. Member of the Therapeutics and Pharmacology Technical Committee.

Richard H. Blum Chairman of the International Research Group for Drug Legislation and Programs. Formerly: Consulting Professor of Psychology, Director, Drug Program, School of Law, Stanford University. Former US delegate to the UN Narcotics Commission.

Kettil Bruun Research Director of the Finnish Foundation for Alcohol Studies, Helsinki.

Allan E. Dyer Assistant Deputy Minister, Ministry of Health, Ontario.

Klaus-Wolf von Eickstedt Director and Professor, Institute for Drugs, Bundesgesundheitsamt, Berlin

Katherine Elliott Assistant Director, The Ciba Foundation, London.

Michael J. Flynn Medical Adviser, TIL (Medical), Ltd. London.

Hans Friebel Chairman, Arzneimittelkommission der Deutschen Aerzteschaft, Cologne.

Gordon R. Fryers Consultant Director of Medical Affairs, Proprietary Association of Great Britain.

Matthew Gwee Senior Lecturer in Pharmacology, University of Singapore.

Notes on Contributors

Elina Hemminki Senior Assistant, Department of Public Health Sciences, University of Tampere, Finland.

Andrew Herxheimer Senior Lecturer in Clinical Pharmacology and Therapeutics, Charing Cross Hospital Medical School, London University. Chairman of Medical Working Group, International Organization of Consumer Unions. Editor, *Drug and Therapeutics Bulletin.*

Jorge Katz Director, IDB/ECLA Research Project on Technology in Latin America (Inter American Development Bank/UN Economic Commission for Latin America), Buenos Aires.

Erich Kaufer Professor of Economics, Institut für Wirtschaftstheorie und Wirtschaftspolitik der Universität Innsbruck.

Kevin Kreitman Assistant in the socio-psycho-pharmacology project, Program in drug and community studies, Stanford University.

Sanjaya Lall Senior Research Officer, Institute of Economics and Statistics, University of Oxford. Consultant for the United Nations Conference for Trade and Development, the UN Industrial Development Organization, the UN Centre on Transnational Corporations, the International Labour Office and the World Bank.

Louis Lasagna Professor of Pharmacology and Toxicology, University of Rochester.

Desmond Laurence Professor of Pharmacology and Therapeutics, School of Medicine, University College, London.

John Lilja Head, Department of Social Pharmacy, Uppsala University.

Wilfred Lionel Associate Professor of Pharmacology, University of Colombo. Secretary, Committee for the Approval of Drugs, Ministry of Health, Sri Lanka.

Alex Lumbroso Managing Director, Laboratoires Manceau SA, Massy, France.

Notes on Contributors

Mia Lydecker Research Associate and Principal Editor, Health Policy Program, School of Medicine, University of California, San Francisco.

Alan Maislisch Formerly: Technology Division, UNCTAD, Geneva.

Neville Milner WHO Pharmacist, Aden, Peoples Democratic Republic of Yemen.

Anne Firth Murray Program Officer, Hewlett Foundation, Palo Alto. Formerly: Health Policy Program, University of California Medical School, San Francisco.

Edith Penrose Professor of Political Economy, Institut Européen d'Administration des Affaires, Fontainebleau.

Georges Peters Professor of Pharmacology, Faculty of Medicine, Lausanne.

Bror Rexed Director of the United Nations Fund for Drug Abuse Control. Formerly: Director, National Board of Health and Welfare, Sweden.

George Rosenkrantz Chairman of the Board, Syntex Corporation, Mexico City.

Malcolm Segall Fellow, Institute for Development Studies, Sussex University.

Milton Silverman Senior Faculty, Health Policy Program. University of California Medical School, San Francisco. Formerly: Special Assistant to the Secretary, Department of Health, Education and Welfare, USA.

Pierre Simon Professor of Clinical Pharmacology, Faculty of Medicine Pitié-Salpêtrière, University of Paris VI.

Peter Schiøler Chief Consultant on Alcohol and Narcotic Problems, Ministry of Education, Denmark.

M.I. Soueif Professor of Psychology, Cairo University.

Notes on Contributors

Catherine Stenzl Coordinator, International Research Group for Drug Legislation and Programs.

Gerry Stimson Senior Lecturer in Sociology, Goldsmith College, University of London.

*Denis Varonos Professor of Pharmacology, University of Athens, Greece.

*Wilma J. Winter Technical Writer, Bureau of Drugs, US Food and Drug Administration.

Jasper Woodcock Director of the Institute for the Study of Drug Dependence, London.

*Teow Seng Yeoh Professor of Pharmacology, University of Singapore.

*John S. Yudkin Locum Consultant Physician, Whittington Hospital, London. Formerly: Lecturer in Metabolism and Endocrinology, London Hospital Medical College, University of London. Formerly: Senior Lecturer in Medicine, Dar-es-Salaam.

*Irving Kenneth Zola Professor of Sociology, Brandeis University, Waltham, Massachusetts.

We wish to affirm the obvious; that commentators and advisers (indicated by *) are not to be held responsible for the content of chapters to which they have rendered assistance, but which may not reflect their opinion.

The final responsibility for all materials rests with the chapter authors and in no instance reflects any official opinion of organisations with which they or any chapter adviser are associated.

FOREWORD

by Dr T.A. Lambo, Deputy Director-General, World Health Organisation

The authors of this book, a group of specialists and experts from diverse backgrounds and nationalities, but having as a common denominator sub-disciplines in the health professions, have addressed themselves succinctly, objectively, and I think brilliantly and effectively to the elucidation of some of the medical issues and data bearing on the major aspects of the process of medicines provision.

The process begins with research in the laboratory, going through manufacture, with drug evaluation, thence through education of prescribers and dispensers, and finally to the central figure, the consuming patient. At each stage there are difficulties, many of which are resolvable should the parties concerned be wise enough to read this book. The authors are strong friends of education in the public interest. This book is itself proof, for it is an education, and a worthy one, for any of us who care about medicines and health, or for that matter national thrift or the expansion of international collaboration.

My commendations are twofold: first, to the editors and authors who have worked so hard and so long in the service of the health of mankind and science, with thrift and common sense; and secondly, to the potential reader, commending this book to him or her. And who is that reader? By my lights the reader will be every government authority anywhere concerned with drug policy, anyone teaching clinical pharmacology, all concerned with cultural or social medicine, or medical economics, and most certainly my own colleagues at every level who attend to international issues and collaboration in health affairs.

PREFACE

The editors, authors and commentators contributing to this book have commitments in common. We believe that improved health care depends on improvements in the provision of medicines. We are aware that the 'system' which begins with drug discovery and has, as its endpoint, a patient's use of a drug is complex and has internal contradictions and conflicts; but, we hold, the 'system' itself can benefit from being studied, by policy revision and the evaluation of the outcome of policy operations. We believe further, that policies and practices must conform to local situations (whether national or regional), and that assessment of these situations rests on adequate research methods — from economics to epidemiology.

We further hold, and this volume is our testimony, that a necessary approach to medicines provision, which is both health-stimulating and economically sensible, is an international affair. This is why we are ourselves an international group, why we recommend international diversity in evaluating the process of medicines provision, and why we are committed to the importance of international bodies as sources of co-ordination, information and assistance.

For the most part, we are oriented here towards what we hope to be the interests of the consumer, and necessarily his or her political self, and the government which is mandated to serve citizen-welfare. Yet we are not unmindful of the important role of industry in the discovery and manufacture of drugs. Whatever the source of capital which is to support pharmacological research and pharmaceutical development, such capital must be available.

Our efforts have been possible only through the good will of our contributors, and the support of governments, private institutions and international agencies and groups. We gratefully acknowledge financial support from the British Department of Health and Social Security, the Danish Ministry of Education, and the Foundation for International Research on Drug Legislation and Control. We are particularly indebted to the Right Honourable David Owen, former Minister of Health and Social Security in the United Kingdom, Dr Peter Schiøler, Chief Consultant on Alcohol and Narcotics Problems to the Danish Ministry of Education, and to the International Organization of Consumer Unions. We are grateful to Maître Robert Turretini, Geneva, Dr Dick Joyce of

CIBA-Geigy (Basle), Nicolaas Bel, Head of the Division of Pharmacy and Economic Legislation in the EEC Commission and to the staff of the WHO Secretariat in Geneva who were all generous with their time and knowledge.

INTRODUCTION

This book is for those authoritatively concerned with the provision of medicines. By the provision of medicines, we mean efforts to achieve an optimal distribution, worldwide, to patients and consumers so as best to assure health. By 'authoritatively' concerned, we mean those people who, by virtue of position or interest, are in a position to do something about medicines' provision. They include: public-health policy administrators, legislators, public-sector economists, research workers in health-service administration and health economics, health-service planners, pharmaceutical industry managers and their associates in marketing, i.e. those who represent professional or consumer interests in relation to drug distribution; and the teachers of physicians, pharmacists and other drug dispensers, together with the journalists who write for consumers.

We speak of medicines, by which we mean all those substances which people seek out or are given with the intention of preventing or treating illness, alleviating symptoms or improving health. The range is wide, from sophisticated modern drugs for rare diseases to over-the-counter remedies for aches and pains; it includes, of course, folk medical preparations, from plants to poultices.

Clearly, not all medicines used today should be used, and others ought to be and are not in use. Thus we speak of 'optimal' and in so-doing quickly reach the heart of the matter. Optimal is ideal, and what is ideal depends upon what people value; how one defines a good or a bad thing, a cost or a benefit. But 'optimal' is also pragmatic: it connotes what can be done. And to know what can be done requires a knowledge of medicines, illnesses, available resources and how people act and are influenced. Optimal also implies an active choice, based not only on knowledge and foresight, but also on planning and, importantly, on making an overt order out of the many possibilities so as to emerge with policies and priorities. To have ideals, to be pragmatic, to be capable, and to order affairs into policy is the business of those whom we call authoritative in health, and it is to that international group this book is addressed.

Why has this book been written? Because the job is not easy and because anyone concerned with the provision of medicines will benefit from up-to-date information about matters which do — or should —

influence decisions. Not that facts are enough, for as noted, much valuing and weighing goes into policy-making, advising and teaching. So we aim to identify major issues that surround the provision of medicines: problems of health priority; economics; under- or over-regulation in drug development, marketing and distribution; prescribing by physicians; and drug use by consumers.

The planning of this volume itself reflects one kind of policy-making. An initial phase of discussion and problem identification went on over many years amongst a group of scientists, physicians, drug producers and public administrators who, as affiliates of the Inter-national Research Group on Drug Legislation and Programs, had first been concerned with the provision and control of psychoactive drugs. During that work, which included the production of a number of papers and books, we became aware of similar issues affecting medicines in general. Amongst our colleagues, employed in public offices, teaching, industry and laboratories, we also met much that we can best call confusion. This is hardly surprising since the issues are complex and rarely set forth dispassionately. As a result of our own increasing awareness, we became convinced that a book which sought to present basic issues and information would be of use.

The next decision had to do with 'how'. Because the Research Group has always been international in membership, in its definition of problems and in its work, we were clear from the start that we had to deal with the provision of medicines worldwide. Such a broad perspective forbade the narrow analysis of problems or facts from only one country or region. It also reaffirmed the need for the contributors and planners of this volume themselves to represent an international array of knowledge and interests. Because the Group had been working effectively together for some years, across frontiers and disciplines, we were also able to draw on some of our own practical experience. We are committed to a style of work which allows all contributors to participate fully and without friction, and to propose solutions to diverse practical problems in a way that can be generally acceptable. The resulting work is empirical.

We understand that this is a world in which ideological differences not only exist but are profoundly important to those who hold particular positions. Thus, one must accept differences, accord those who differ the same respect accorded to those with whom one agrees ideologically, and finally, not aim at general consensus, but simply the agreeable illumination of differences as such, with the presentation of the options inherent in each. An option, of course, is a choice with an estimated outcome. Therefore, we present options when we can, derived from considered values, estimating outcomes based on such projections as can be made from empirical data.

In communicating with each other about this book — and to those institutions and governments who supported the work — we have stressed our intent (which is an expression of the Group's working style) not to espouse a particular policy to the exclusion of others and not to address the problems of one region to the exclusion of others. Each participant has, instead, agreed to seek those facts he can, sort out the issues which seem most salient, and offer various possibilities to the reader; these options are accompanied whenever possible by empirically based estimates of impact, cost and benefit. In each instance, where recommendations are made, the diversity of settings around the world is kept in mind.

The choice of action always belongs to those responsible. In the case of an individual who has authority in relation to the provision of medicines, no group of advisers can be so wise as to know the particulars of a setting or the imperatives of a history. The contributors to this book, more distant than ordinary advisers, will know less of local matters even if they have sought to know more of the general world of fact which bears on their special field. These facts compel us not to be dogmatic but, contrariwise, to offer an array of data and choices; the choice of subsequent action is left to the reader, as it always is, anyway.

With this theme, how did we come to our contributors? It is a big world, and none of us acquainted with it all, not even with all of those sharing our professional activities, however specialised the area. Given the Group's initial commitment to international representation of interests and skills, we could only proceed as people usually do, down a chain of acquaintance and recommendation. The only uniform standard imposed is professional integrity. Our other standards imposed diversity; for example, we wished to be sure that qualified persons from countries at different technological levels of development participated. We had to be sure that differing orientations and diverse geographical regions were represented. Interest by vocational identity is also important; the view of medicines policies from the university, government, clinic, consumer group or pharmaceutical industry can be diverse enough to require that all contribute.

The aim is not a pot-pourri but a blend of experience, perspective and reason. That aim dictated the method by which the book was constructed. First, an international group discussed and agreed upon the format, these discussions going on over several years. With the format fixed and the authors of each chapter agreed, the group helped the authors achieve a fair balance by circulating each chapter to an appropriate panel of commentators. However, the final responsibility for the text as published rests with the individual authors.

Let us look at some of the major themes which emerge. First of all the providing of medicine invokes the very serious interest of groups who, in the present scheme of things, must come to disparate solutions, because of their ideals, duties, self-interest and diverse cultural histories. A regulator, who sees his job as one of ensuring primarily safety, cannot agree with a researcher who sees his job as discovery, or a seller or advertiser who seeks to maximise profit. A physician, hard pressed to see 100 patients a day and under a felt demand from all to 'give me something' will not be patient with the clinical pharmacologist, critical of overprescribing, or the health economist worried about over-expenditure on medicines. A specialist in rare diseases will want public funds spent on medicines to treat 'his' ailment — so will his patients — but the finance authorities in a country (or health or hospital system) with much illness and little money will give a different priority to medicines research, purchase and distribution. It is thus clear that where there is competition for resources or dispute over priorities and procedures, the provision of medicines will be a matter of debate.

Generally, when important affairs are not agreed upon, there will be several immediate results. One is dissatisfaction with the way things are; another is the attempt to exercise power to achieve one solution over another; a third is bargaining, trade-offs and compromise, and a fourth is a sense of confusion among non-experts, along with a real instability in policy. If one adds to these reactions the contribution of actual change, in this instance, new drugs, new knowledge, revised aspirations, and changes in resource availability (some places, systems and people get poorer, some get richer), then instability increases. We believe that in much of the world there is instability in medicines policy, including what is taught to physicians about prescribing or what is told to con-sumers. For that reason alone, since instability implies the opportunity for planned change as well as the inevitability of change itself, this book may be of some assistance.

A second theme is related to what medicines are for. That ought to be simple enough — and it can be, providing one attends to abstract definitions rather than to what medicines or people really do. Con-ventionally, medically 'officially' so to speak, medicines are used to cure illness, as replacement or maintenance therapies, to relieve symptoms, or to prevent disorder. But the intent with which a medicine is used may not achieve the stated aim, or it may do so only partially, or it may create unwanted effects at the same time (side effects, adverse reactions, etc.). These common difficulties are discussed under the rubrics of 'safety' (or toxicity), 'efficacy', or in terms of 'indications' and 'contra-indications'; when one is talking about either minor ills or minor medicines, one contrasts 'trivial' with 'non-trivial' compounds. None of these considerations is all or none; most substances or situations arrange themselves on a continuum, and the continuum shifts depending upon the variables at hand (characteristics of the patient, illness, environment, manner of administration, dosage, repetition of dose, etc.). Troublesomely, each such consideration can be independent, or as in the case of safety and efficacy, there may be regular inverse correlations; as one goes up, the other goes down.

The conflicts caused by the simultaneous operation of several aims, which may be reflected in using several criteria for estimating the goodness or badness of a medicine, mean that there will be many situations — in drug development and regulation or in prescribing or consumer use — where no ideal solution is at hand. Whatever one does, something will be wrong with it. Whoever it is whose body hurts, or whose regulatory agency is accused, or whose product is challenged, or whose money is wasted, will measure the outcome by the standards most relevant to him. This puts people and institutions in conflict: judging the same act, they reach different conclusions as to whether the act (production, regulation, prescribing, etc.) was good or bad. This is not to say there can be no agreement about medicines; it is to say that there can be no agreement unless people agree not simply on definitions but on priorities as well. Sometimes yes, sometimes no; in the foreseeable future conflicts will continue. Contributors to this book hope that illumination of complexities and a factual review will enable providers of medicine to discuss differences objectively and, in some cases, even to achieve consensus.

The functions of medicines are not limited to the demonstrable, conventional medical effects mentioned above. A drug manufacturer marketing a useless or dangerous product; an advertiser defining as an 'indication' a non-illness situation (a mother crying as her child goes off to school for the first day, and the advertisement saying she is 'depressed' and needs a powerful anti-depressant drug); a physician prescribing in lieu of taking time to diagnose or talk to a patient; a consumer buying laxatives so as to be 'regular' twice a day; a politician promoting the use of an ineffective product because a contingent of his constituents advocate it; or a health bureaucrat using medicines policy as a lever for his promotion; these are all examples of functions of medicines. And each is problematic.

As one begins to look at what people do, as opposed to the 'formal' standards for rationality, as these are set forth by experts, one detects a vast new set of functions for medicines, i.e. 'indications' for use, and criteria by which use or outcomes are observed. Consider that just 'doing something' is often important in times of worry or crisis, or that, as in folk practices, one seeks control by expressing wishes or intentions, manipulating words and materials in culturally approved magical rituals. Consider that for physicians some of the therapeutic gain from drugs is via the placebo effect — not much removed from magic — or that what goes on when family members give one another medicines is an expression of interest, affection and/or anxiety on the part of the giver, and appreciation, obedience or relief of worry on the part of the medicine taker.

These examples should suffice to expose the gulf between a formal view of medicinal functions and the psychological and social functions on the part of dispensers and users. Dramatic conflicts rarely emerge (except with the psychoactive drugs, as for example when marijuana users are called criminals) because the advocates of the formal system are usually in power, whereas folk users and doers are not. Ordinary people when confronted may deny or rationalise their conduct so as to conform to a more 'rational' or expert external standard. The problem is, nevertheless, that medicines policy cannot easily be implemented until one knows what people are really doing and why, how to reach them to educate them (whether doctors or patients), and what 'irrational' substitute conduct to expect in advance, should one remove a substance without providing a replacement for it in a specific function. A pragmatist will attend to such issues; they constitute the real world.

The question arises, how far can medicines policy be planned? How many plans can be implemented? One can, of course, always create new bureaucracies to spend money, to issue regulations, to intrude on commerce, medicine, folk and family life, but what justifies it? Immensely important issues arise here. One has to do with concepts of the ideal role of the state; how much regulation is desired? How much safety is the state expected to guarantee for citizens; how honest is such a guarantee, given nature's surprises and the frailty of life? One also asks about the evidence for success when plans are administered which affect medical care and personal efforts to seek health and relieve pain. At what cost to other sectors does one gain improvements and where does the curve of increasing inefficiency begin its upward slope? How good are planners and policy-makers; what kinds of problems respond to their measures and which do not? Or, if one looks at how medicinal health care can be influenced, can one be sure that a policy will use the working levers it does have, instead of others that policy-makers may be more used to pulling?

There is also the question of medicines *vis-à-vis* the larger context of health care; how important is it to attend to medicines given other demands affecting health levels, e.g. nutrition, pollution, sanitation, population growth, traffic accidents, knowledge about self-care, the prevalence of disease vectors, or the extent of medical resources *per se*? Were one to include those aspects of mental health affected if not determined by the social environment, then the array of factors influencing health becomes even broader, and the role of medicines — however important — remains rather narrow and specific as a component of health care competing for priority. This concreteness is, of course, an advantage. One can do something about materials; it may be more difficult to influence the general environment.

To identify factors affecting health, and subsequently to allocate resources for preventive or remedial work, requires a clear idea of what one means by 'health'. That is not simply a matter of constructing an abstract definition; perhaps there can be agreement on ideals. The job is to learn what the operational definitions are which, day-to-day, lead a person to wonder if he might be ill, or cause a physician to make or withhold a diagnosis. Health definitions of the sort people live by are embedded in cultural concepts, ideas about how life is maintained, pain avoided or death fended off. In pluralist societies there will be competing notions and practices in health maintenance. These differences will be reflected in what people think of drugs and how they use them.

In Western societies there is an awkward mind/body dichotomy and a technological bent which leads many trained in medicine to concentrate on 'real medical practice', brushing aside the substance of social medicine or mental health as irrelevant or soft-headed. If the 'real' business of medicine is limited to pain, microbes, tissue pathology, viruses and the like, then medicines policy might be restricted likewise. To do so is impossible, for if one examines the purpose of use of medicines which account for the lion's share of prescriptions or self-medication in the same technological societies, it will be seen that the consumption of psychoactive drugs is foremost, these ranging from alcohol or aspirin to diazepam. Thus, what people are mostly medicating is something in their heads. But the problem is not just in how people feel, it is in how communities and politicians feel as well, for psychoactive substances account for the single most difficult area in drug policy, that of 'drug abuse'. That problem is not discussed in this volume, but it is noted here to illustrate a conflict central to much in medicines policy: the fact that what people do with drugs may not be what others think is best for them.

Even if one were to focus on 'real' medical practice alone, cultural and psychological factors would still be important. Essential aspects of public health are the life-styles and belief systems which express what ordinary people do to stay or get well, or which have been identified, by scientific methods, as behaviours with a major influence on health levels. These range from the relatively simple matters of 'compliance' – do people take the drugs prescribed for them? – to nutrition, sanitation, risk exposure and the like. Consider, for example, that the initial breakthroughs in disease prevention have, historically, occurred not through the application of medical scientific knowledge, but in sanitation (see Dubos, 1959).

Consider the current evidence for the importance of the citizen's own habits in the prevention of recovery from cardio-vascular disease: avoiding overweight, cigarettes, excess alcohol, and securing a balanced diet and enough exercise. Consider, too, the accumulating data suggesting that many diseases are precipitated by manufacturing technology, for example, carcinogenic products and by-products. Since what people do may largely determine their health status, authorities concerned with public health need to become folk-oriented, to understand what motivates people's conduct and how to influence it and certainly that applies to the use of medicines by consumers, be their role that of patients or self-medicators.

Engel (1977) has suggested that scientific medicine has become, for the West, 'the dominant folk model of disease'. That model, technical and reductionist in its biomedical (molecular biological) emphasis, stands in contrast to the folk criteria which people use in making judgements about being ill. Those criteria are primarily psychological, social, cultural – how people feel, look and act. No wonder then that so many of the drugs – and related products such as cosmetics, vitamins, etc. – which people use are directed to changing how one feels, looks or acts. To that list, one adds preparations that are intended to change how people smell, eliminate, sleep, smile, perform sexually, etc.

Prompting the use of drugs then is the desire for an immediate effect on those aspects of a person's feelings and performance which are immediately accessible to his own senses or values. When these efforts do not work, when the person does not know what is wrong, or when the folk and medical criteria for defining illness are the same, then people go to the doctor or other healer.

Although these criteria can coincide, it is safer to assume that there are two belief systems about health in societies where the scientific medical view is held. There is the formal, technical or intellectual health system. In contrast to it stands the informal or folk health belief system, which includes its own 'pharmacology', i.e. what substances are good for what conditions and when and how much is to be taken. These beliefs are part of family and group lore and determine how individuals use many medicaments. To the extent that citizens are educated to the technological contents of scientific medicine, the overlap between folk systems and technical ones increases so that an increasing portion of what people do is what a physician might have them do — if the doctor himself was a 'pure' medical scientist and not also a creature of his own folk culture and personal idiosyncrasies. The elements may explain some of the great variability between physicians cross-culturally and some of the differences between professionals within a society. One should not assume, of course, that wisdom comes only from technical medicine, that pharmacological education always flows from an intellectual élite to the masses. The history of pharmacology tells us otherwise; witness the use in the folk culture of compounds such as aspirin, rauwolfia, digitalis, opium, etc., and their adoption in technical medicine.

The existence of two systems, technical and folk (which interrelate to some extent), implies two levels of control for health and health care. One is governed by the day-to-day habits and judgements of ordinary people. The other is 'expert', consisting of medical professionals with their allied disciplines and institutions. When people become sick enough to come into hospital, it is the 'expert' system which controls them entirely. As outpatients, the expert system tells them what to do and what to take. When people are going about their ordinary lives, not seeing doctors, the expert system has little direct contact with them, except that it may offer information and advice through the media.

The 'expert' system does affect ordinary folk indirectly, for it also constitutes a bureaucracy. Bureaucracies arise whenever knowledge is specialised and carries with it attributes of power. The expert bureaucracy, in most countries, spends most of its time trying to influence individual health indirectly by shaping events or products which, in turn, affect lives. Only those bureaucracies which are in direct contact with citizens, as for example, those formulating and delivering health information or primary health care, avoid the need to work at a distance from the consumer. An example of the expert system working at a distance — where the locus of control is well beyond the individual citizen affected, for whom the system purportedly is run — is the regulation of the provision of medicines.

Controls which are exercised by individuals as 'folk', are highly efficient; no one is in a better condition to govern the time and amount of medicines used — or exercise or smoking, etc. — than the person himself. Efficiency here also implies low cost; no taxpayer pays for an institution to provide experts or servants to supervise or perform these functions for the citizen. But health control exercised by oneself — or in the family — is deficient as well as efficient; for insofar as the individual lacks resources — knowledge, money, skills, opportunities, to act in a way which optimises health, the result will be less than optimal.

The 'expert' on the other hand (for example, the bureaucrat in charge of a health service or regulatory system) inevitably has more resources in terms of knowledge, money and facilities, for he draws on institutional and national funds, knowledge, personnel and services. While he may not be able to optimise his functions because of actual limits on his access to those resources, the bureaucrat can always develop an ideal plan which represents what he 'would' do if he had all possible resources and if his aspirations — based on knowledge and values of what 'could' be — became his objectives.

The actual work of any bureaucrat is very inefficient, however, because what he seeks to control, do or affect is always removed from himself, the actual performance being vested in other people, units or institutions. Furthermore much of what other people are doing, which he seeks to influence, is often work performed for others still: e.g. the laboratory technician testing a drug; the clerk filing a report on drug effects; the copywriter writing a drug advertisement, etc. Necessarily, the work is ultimately influenced by competing forces, e.g. instructions of a work supervisor, regulations imposed by another bureaucrat in another agency, or the worker's own interests and perspectives. (Perhaps the worker would rather go fishing than check that the device which counts x number of pills into bottles is functioning accurately.)

Inefficiency implies a high cost. There can be little question that the greater the intended span of the bureaucrat's influence — the more activities in more places — the higher the loss and variability which, to counterbalance and correct, requires greater expenditure of energy, funds, typewriter ribbons, etc. Reports, supervision, assistants, inspection, repetition and threat all become devices to improve the efficiency of a bureaucrat, so that he may better influence a product or an act which, in turn, somewhere down the line is presumed to affect a citizen as patient/consumer. Furthermore, unless one does research on impact one cannot, of course, be sure that the ultimate effect will be the one the bureaucrat intends. Does an informational label on a medicine bottle get read? Is it understood? Does understanding lead to safer home use? Should the medicine have been prescribed in the first place?

What a bureaucrat does is to implement a policy. Whether he exists or, existing, does anything at all depends on whether or not there *is* a policy with instructions and resources allocated to implement it. Three essential questions bear on whether or not there *should* be medicines policies. Can they be made efficient without undue cost? Will policies achieve the health effects at the consumer/patient level which are intended? Are we sure those 'intentions' reflect primarily the best interests of the consumer? Good policy-making implies: that alternative goals have been considered; that the objectives decided upon are clear; that means for achieving them are known; and that methods for measuring the cost of implementation and actual impact are put to use.

The foregoing constitute the minimal requirements for a rational medicines policy. Implicit is the earlier point, that one know what one means by health. One also needs to know the relationship of the medicines under consideration to health, and one should have weighed the priorities for competing influences on health.

The concept of a rational policy for the provision of medicines assumes that there is sufficient knowledge to know what to do. When that is the case, the answer to the question 'Can medicines policy be rationalised?' is yes. But even then knowledge alone is not sufficient. To rationalise policy also implies that one has intrinsic order in a society — also in the minds of policy planners and executors — and that such order can be furthered through planning. The notion of order as essential to planning also indicates that conflict is subordinated, that is, the diverse and competing interests of politics, profit, professional power and diverse cultural beliefs about health are sufficiently mellowed to allow first creative debate and then consensus on what is to be done. Conflict can, of course, be suppressed when power is sufficient, be that the power of argument based on knowledge or simple political clout. The imposition of the latter is always costly. Yet power has, to date, always been required whenever there is a medicines policy to be implemented.

The question, whether or not the costs of using power offset its negative effects, is essential in considering whether it is worth trying to rationalise medicines policy. The criteria are political and economic and will differ according to the values of a given society. But, whenever there is a governmental plan which is to be imposed on some aspect of the development, production, distribution, dispensing or consumption of medicines, one of the side-effects will be a fiscal cost to the population. Another side effect will be that some people will have to do things they do not want to do (or refrain from doing what they want to do). A consumer may not like a safety-capped bottle; a cancer patient may want to take a forbidden medicine; a pharmacist may wish to sell a drug but cannot do so without a doctor's order, or a manufacturer might wish to market a drug without governmental clearance. To the extent that a policy will intrude on people's habits or interests, or create circumstances where previously optional conduct — or products — are newly forbidden, the costs of having a policy will be infringements on others. Such infringements, in the service of the larger public good, are part of the business of governments. The essence of a medicines policy is to decide when they are justified and worth the cost.

If one examines existing medicines policies, nationally and internationally, one will find that they cover or address at least the following areas:

Economics. Is the provision of medicines (invention, production, distribution, consumption) to be profit or non-profit; state or private; if a profit industry, with controlled or uncontrolled profits; taxed or not taxed? Are consumers to pay or receive drugs free? Who pays the costs and how? If any aspect of medicine provision is to be regulated, who pays the costs? What are the direct and indirect costs of regulation?

Developing and Introducing Drugs. How does this work and how is it supported? What rules govern inventive and developmental work? Are there priorities for drug development? What standards are applied to decide whether the work is done well? Who makes those judgements?

How are regulatory powers enforced?

Marketing and Distribution. Who markets and distributes drugs? Are there regulations on what drugs shall be available? Are priorities assigned as to what shall be more or less available? How accurately and completely are drugs described? Where are they described? Who is allowed to buy, hold or re-distribute drugs? Who can dispense, prescribe, recommend or advertise medicines to consumers? Along the marketing chain, are there regulations governing purity, profits, quantity supplied, containers, storage conditions, records, security? How are regulations enforced?

Regulating Bodies. How are these constituted? What are their powers and whence are they derived? Who funds and staffs them? Who supervises them, assesses their efficiency and impact? How do their rules and operations get changed?

Professional Conduct. Who decides what physicians, pharmacists, nurses and paramedical personnel may do with medicines? Who sets the standards for qualifying personnel in these and other health roles with responsibility for distribution and administration of medicines? Is there to be supervision of what is done? How is supervision performed and enforced? Do regulations govern what responsible personnel must know about medicines? Who has responsibility for teaching and informing? Are there standards which govern the quality of that information?

Consumers. Are there regulations governing what patients/consumers may or may not do with drugs in their possession? What provisions are made to assure consumer access to medicines and information about medicines? What provisions prevent access to medicines or information? What agencies have responsibility for assessing patient/consumer needs, problems or conduct? How are resources allocated to assure information about consumer interests and needs? Who pays?

International Bodies. Which international bodies have been created and what are their duties with respect to medicines? How are these duties performed and co-ordinated? Who pays for these services? What assessments are made of international needs relating to medicines provision?

The foregoing list — a limited one which does little justice to wide national differences – gives little attention to the direct education of consumers (patients or clients) so as to bring health control closer to them, who are after all potentially the most efficient supervisors of their own health care. Perhaps experts in general and their bureaucracies perform like the physicians whom Pratt, Seligman and Reader (1958) studied. They thought very little of their patients' interest or ability to learn, and the less highly they regarded their clients the less they told them. In almost all cases, professionals told their clients very little about the whys and hows of their illnesses or of the doctor's recommendations and prescriptions.

There has been very little reason in the past to be sanguine about health education in schools; some research has indicated it did not work. More recent studies, notably Maccoby and Farquhar (1975) and Blum *et al.* (1976) suggest that consumer health education can have some impact. The task is to find the most auspicious situations, methods, vehicles and audiences for a positive educational impact.

The growth of the consumer movement has prompted interest in informing consumers. Its emphasis has been on the quality of goods and services rendered commercially or by government. More recently 'consumerism' has begun to examine the quality of professional services as well, including what physicians do. An important feature of consumer-oriented work is skepticism, a readiness to doubt whether products or services are as they are claimed to be. When applied to dispensing practices and medicines, that scepticism looks critically at the claims – and the systems of belief and service – of physicians and drug producers. What is good for doctor, druggist or pharmaceutical manufacturer may not be good for the patient as consumer, no matter how golden the providing angel's halo is painted. A corresponding aspect of consumerism is service and product evaluation, i.e. to describe costs and benefits and assess quality.

Implicit in consumerism is the reorganisation of decision-making, particularly the decision as to 'what is good for you'. The tenets of consumerism are (1) rationalism – that humans act wisely when informed; (2) responsibility – that people are individually accountable for what they do, be they suppliers of goods or of services; and (3) advocacy.

Advocacy implies that the interests of the consumer are often not the same as the interests of those who are paid by the consumer (whether directly as in free-market economies, or via taxation or increased product costs as in nationalised or socialist health services) to serve or supply him. Conflict of interest is assumed to exist as is the need to act aggressively through legitimate channels in order to further consumer interests.

Consumer protection is sought through insisting on information, that is, requiring providers of goods and services to reveal data about process, cost and quality. When there is evidence of extensive deficiencies in quality, or unreasonable cost, the effort is to institute quality and cost controls by either institutional self-policing or governmental authority. When deficient services are government activities, the conflict between consumers and the bureaucracy expresses itself through judicial (in nations where these are available remedies) and political processes. Each of these defences or aspiration-advancing steps depends in part upon the availability and dissemination of information. For that reason, this book seeks to present material of potential value to consumer advocates.

We come now to the final emphasis which characterises this book. It is the belief that the provision of medicines is not only a worldwide interest, but that it requires co-ordinated international activities in the public interest. The nature of those activities — fact-finding, policy consideration and implementation — is suggested by this introductory chapter. What now requires affirmation is our belief that sufficient data are at hand to demonstrate that it is appropriate to exchange information and develop international standards by which to judge several of the steps in the provision of medicines.

The world offers a natural laboratory in which to observe diverse practices and policies in medicines provision. Information from that laboratory deserves to be widely shared. That implies an impetus to further cross-national research, to further exchanges among academics, administrators, consumers, and to the enhancement of facilities for observation, information exchange and policy evaluation. Our conviction that a world view is instructive, and that worldwide information exchange is necessary, have set both the format and the emphasis of this book. Like the World Health Organisation's current efforts, it is a beginning.

References

Blum, R.H., Blum, E. and Garfield, E. (1976). *Drug Education: Results and Recommendations*, Lexington, Mass., Lexington Books

Dubos, R. (1959). *Mirage of Health*, New York, Harper & Row

Engel, G.L. (1977). The need for a new medical model: a challenge for biomedicine. *Science 196*, 129-36

Maccoby, N. and Farquhar, J.W. (1975). Communication for health. Unselling heart disease. *J. Commun 25* (3), Summer, 114-26

Pratt, L. Seligman, A. and Reader, G.G. (1958) Physicians' views on the level of medical information among patients. In *Patients, Physicians and Illness*, Ill., Glencoe, 222-8

1 MEDICINES – THE INTERESTED PARTIES

Jasper Woodcock

Medicines are a focus of powerful economic, social, and emotional forces. While their contribution to the improvement of health and increase of life expectancy is said to be small compared to that of sanitation and other public health measures (McKeown, 1979), their impact as alleviators of suffering, curers of individual ills, relievers of your or my symptom, gives their provision a significance to the individual person that other positive measures to improve health can rarely possess. Consider that yesterday we felt ill whereas today, thanks, we believe, to some medicament, we are restored to health. By contrast, the lengthening of our individual lives as a result of hygienic sewage disposal or universal compulsory vaccination against smallpox is not an event we can experience. We know personally the illnesses from which we try, by individual prophylactic measures, to preserve ourselves, but we can make no such experiential connection between our health and longevity and public hygiene. In consequence, public and popular concern about health imbue medicines and those who provide them with an exceptional degree of significance (which the latter may in turn exploit).

In its simplest, ancient form, the provision of medicines might involve only two actors – the healer (whether shaman, priest or herbalist) and the patient. The prototypical medicine is likely to have been a herb endowed with real or attributed curative powers or perhaps some other natural object rendered potent by the healer's manipulation, as for example an amulet. Hippocrates, Galen and Dioscorides themselves prepared the medicines they prescribed. When the forerunner of the present day pharmacy appeared, the apothecary's shop, this did not so much represent a division between the processes of diagnosis/prescription and the supply of medicines as the appearance of a rival profession claiming equally with wizards, priests, physicians and surgeons the power and the wherewithal to heal. The potency of the medicament was interdependent with the authority of the prescriber. It would have been meaningless for a patient to have questioned what his doctor prescribed as something separable from his doctor's competence (the remnants of this state of affairs can still be discerned in the attitude of many doctors!). It might be truer then to say that in the prototypical provision of medicines there is only one actor, the doctor/prescriber; the patient, as the word suggests, is a passive consumer.

Today, patients are increasingly being encouraged to become active participants in the process. Popular pharmacopoeias, such as those by Pradal (1974) or Parish (1979) are being published to enable patients to discuss their medication knowledgeably with their doctors. But this is a recent development in a historical process, under which a number of intermediaries have entered into the transaction between medicine prescriber and medicine taker.

Consider them all: the industry which produces medicines; another industry which produces quite related products psychologically – the 'health food' sector; the governmental regulatory authorities; international agencies concerned with drugs; governmental or other institutional purchasing authorities; medical-pharmacological research workers; medical sales representatives; private insurers; retail and clinical pharmacists; physicians themselves; and finally, the patient – perhaps as part of a family – who, *qua* consumer, may also be represented by consumer organisations. Add to these direct participants in the provision of medicine, their important ancillaries or supervisors, for instance the legislators who write drug control or commercial laws, politicians who define issues in health care, academicians whose research bears on medicines policy (economists, medical anthropologists, public health professors, etc.) and even the news and advertising media whose awareness and handling of medicine-related issues, claims and facts may contribute to public education, outcry, or bamboozlement.

In terms of the theme of this book, the most significant of these intermediaries is the *pharmaceutical industry*. Nowadays the medicines with which we are concerned are almost exclusively the fruits of that industry's research and development and the product of its factories. The present-day industry has its origins firstly in the nineteenth century wholesale druggist and patent remedy business and secondly in the chemical, and particularly the dyestuffs, industry. It is dominated by multinational corporations with a collective reputation for rationalising, economically, and, some would insist, exploiting to the utmost, the utilities inherent in multinational operations and legal status. This is partly in response to the extensive controls imposed by *regulatory authorities* set up in every country seeking to ensure minimum standards of safety and purity, if not efficacy, in pharmaceutical products.

Of course national taxation and price control policies also shape choices made by the international drug companies. The manoeuvrings of the multinational pharmaceutical corporations to avoid restrictions on the use of their products and the populations on which they may be tested, to maximise their profits, and to minimise the taxes paid on them, have been – often indignantly – documented in recent years (UNCTAD, 1975; Haslemere, 1976; Levinson, 1974). Though competition within the industry is keen, it can also sometimes be a sham (Anon., 1976). In any event, there is sufficient identity of interest among individual producers to lead to the establishment of strong national associations to negotiate with the governmental regulatory authorities and, in those countries where state health services are major purchasers of medicines, with *government purchasing agencies*.

There are no internationally sanctioned controls apart from those vested in the International Narcotics Control Board which monitors international trade in drugs likely to create problems because of their potential for non-medical and/or addictive use. While a number of other *international organisations*, such as the World Health Organisation (WHO) and the United Nations Conference on Trade and Development (UNCTAD) have taken a great deal of interest in the provision of medicines (see Chapter 8), none of them are endowed with powers that could limit the ability of the multinationals to exploit their markets, or to assure quality of care standards for prescribing doctors or dispensing pharmacists in the diversely constituted nations of the world. As international control efforts have increased – for example, via the Psychotropic Convention which has brought under the supervision of the International Narcotics Control Board many psychoactive drugs (which have high profit potentials for manufacturers and pharmacists but may damage the consumer, e.g. barbiturates or amphetamines) – so too have efforts to limit impacts on the industry: witness the acquisition of consultative status at the UN for the International Federation of Pharmaceutical Manufacturers.

The absence of effective international organs to control such abusive multinational operations as exist has led some to argue that the most appropriate way to control their power is through multinational *trade unions*, in the case of medicines, through the International Federation of Chemical and General Workers (Levinson, 1974). In practice, however, except insofar as unions may affect medicines' availability through negotiations for health insurance benefits, the unions have had little influence up to now.

The pharmaceutical industry is constantly searching in its own research laboratories for new drugs and, indeed, this is where most new drug discoveries occur. Some of this research is in pursuit of genuinely new compounds but much of it results only in variations of existing drugs which may have marginal advantages over competing products and, equally important, do not infringe rival patents. Once a promising product has been found, however, the manufacturer has to recruit the support of others to test its clinical safety and efficacy. Consequently, the pharmaceutical industry supports a great deal of research carried out by *clinical, medical and pharmacological departments* in hospitals and universities. The requirements of government regulatory agencies have led in some instances to pharmaceutical companies setting up research facilities in places where suitable 'captive' populations are readily available on which to test new drugs, such as prisons in rich countries and 'health centres' in poor ones. Further clinical research relies on physicians in ordinary practices, some of whom are also supported to conduct the later stages of drug trials on their patients. A special problem here is that standards for research design and execution may be inadequate.

As will already be evident, governments have been compelled to establish substantial bureaucracies to regulate the provision of medicines. In some nations these have grown in step not simply with the increasing complexity and sophistication of the pharmaceutical industry's products, but also with a by now worldwide awareness of the ill effects which medicines can bring about. A simple list is a reminder of the fact that almost any medicine or treatment strong enough to be effective is also going to have 'side effects', that is unintended effects which may be dangerous. We need only remember thalidomide, chloramphenicol, diethylstilboestrol, phenacetin. In this sense every medicine is potentially dangerous.

At the beginning, in the nineteenth century it was felt sufficient to channel the supply of potentially poisonous substances through professionally qualified chemists, then later to make some of them available only against a doctor's prescription: neither of these controls required much manpower to enforce. With the introduction of biological substances like vaccines and antisera, inspection and approval of manufacturing techniques and installations became necessary. The present requirements for licensing of new drugs, that of demonstrated safety and therapeutic efficacy, following in the wake of the Stalinon and thalidomide tragedies, have required the expansion of powers of government agencies like the massive US Food and Drug Administration and the smaller UK Medicines Commission.

In countries where the government is a major purchaser of medicines, there can be strong pressure for government agencies to demand not only that the medicines on the market should be safe and effective but also that they should be *necessary*. By that is meant that a new drug (which is frequently a combination of several substances) contributes to health in a way existing products do not. For it is the case that many products are marketed only because their manufacturers seek a competitive product. The wide variation in the number of medicinal products (in the UK called 'medical specialities') marketed in one country in contrast to another suggests wide variations in the stringency with which the criterion of necessity is applied (Dukes and Lunde, 1979). Variations in medicines availability also strongly reflect the varying health needs, adequacy of medical services and, in terms of availability to individuals at low income levels, economic development of nations and regions. Sweden and Denmark manage with between 2000 and 3000 distinct medical specialities, while the UK and Germany have 15,000 at least. (That this is not just a function of population size is attested by Luxembourg's 7,300.) In contrast to these ample numbers, consider that WHO (1979) offers a basic list of only 200-odd essential drugs. WHO argues that not many more than these will supply most of the needs for primary health care in less developed countries.

So long, however, as medicines are manufactured by a competitive pharmaceutical industry, a formidable apparatus of marketing exists to promote their sales. Besides the usual sales promotion methods of advertisements in professional journals and mailing of advertising literature through the post, the provision of medicines occupies a vast army of *sales representatives* throughout the world. The proportion of representatives to physicians varies widely between countries, being as high as one representative for every three or four doctors in countries such as Brazil and Mexico to one in 18 in the UK and one in 32 for Norway (Hemminki and Personen, 1977).

In pharmaceutical marketing the target of salesmanship is the prescribing doctor and not the purchasers of medicines. This has been so because in medically well-served nations, the doctor is the 'gate-keeper', determining what medicines a patient buys or a hospital maintains in its dispensary. The purchasers are either the patients themselves, *private medical insurance schemes*, or where there is a national health scheme, the state. The absence of direct economic links between the doctor who decides what shall be prescribed and *the retail pharmacist* who supplies it to the patient has also tended to delay the emergence of consumerism in the provision of medicines. Recently *consumers' unions* have begun to encourage patients to adopt a more active and questioning role, which of course requires education of the patient as well as confidence in the doctor.

Emphasis on the key role of the doctor as prescriber, however, must not allow us to overlook that there are many compounds which the patient buys without prescription – the over-the-counter remedies (OTCs) such as aspirin, laxatives, antacids, etc. – or what are provided in a family setting in the form of teas, broths, poultices or, in some cultures, magical potions and spells. It should also be remembered that while the doctor may prescribe – or for the hospitalised patient the nurse may offer – the consumer often does determine quite significantly the manner of use of what is prescribed. It is the rule not the exception that patients deviate from their prescription instructions (amount, frequency, duration, etc.) (Stimson, 1974).

At this point it is well to remind ourselves that however narrowly medicines are defined by pharmacologists or government regulators, there are a very wide range of substances which are used *as if* they were medicines, i.e. they have the functions outlined in Chapter 2. Health foods are a major example, enjoying large retail sales in wealthy countries. Some of these 'health' foods are, like other medicines, inherently dangerous; others may become poisonous as a function of their production, e.g. from toxic agricultural sprays or uncontrolled food manufacture.

The food industry – and food advertising – is playing an increasing role in public health concepts; in the US in 1980 the National Institutes of Health offered a list of food 'do's' and 'don'ts' (eat more fibre, less cholesterol, more vegetables, less meat, drink some alcohol but not more than . . . etc.). The issues and factors affecting medicines provision will be similar to those in the food and beverage industry at large. One sees parallels, for example, in the US labelling requirements with respect to mineral, calorie, carbohydrate, vitamin, etc. content of foods and beverages.

Having now identified the major parties whose interests affect the provision of medicines, one can see that conflict as well as diversity of interests are characteristic and, further, motives – when they are ascertainable – may be complex. Patients of course ought to have as their primary interest health, and their role as consumers of medicines would be expected to reflect just a motivation to stay well or recover from illness; but, as an increasing number of observations suggest, medicines may signify love or value-received or a continuing relationship with a doctor rather than health. Furthermore, some patients seem not to want to 'get well'. It certainly should be the case that economic interests would guide patients to seek inexpensive and efficacious medicines, but this also may prove incorrect – in spite of the rational assumptions of consumer organisations. When medicines are free, as in some national health systems, motives of thrift do not appear, and as we all see from advertising successes with OTC compounds, cosmetics, cigarettes or health foods, the product the consumer 'wants' may be both expensive and either useless or harmful.

As for the other actors in the drama, one must attend to more than their public roles and mandates to assess their actual intentions and interests in medicines provision. Regulators, for example (in the US well-known for their tardiness in licensing new drugs) may have more than optimal cost/benefit risk analyses guiding them. A bureaucrat's constituency may well be other than the public – in some countries indeed it may be the pharmaceutical industry itself which calls the tune. Elsewhere, typically bureaucratic self-protection from political outcries may dictate that, in order to avoid any accusations of dangerous drugs having been licensed, the safest course is to license none. Pharmacists too have a split role – as retail businessmen interested in sales on the one hand, and as professionals safeguarding customers from unwise drug usage on the other. Physicians may be assumed only to interest themselves in patient welfare, but that easy surmise is contradicted by evidence that, when pressed to see many patients over a short time, overprescribing is a convenient solution to the problem. Also, with patients – as with gift exchanges in peasant cultures – a repeat prescription may reflect a commitment to a continuing doctor-patient tie, not to wise pharmacotherapy.

Purchasing institutions – whether state health services or group insurance hospitals – should be reliable for their interests in thrift and efficacy. But again this may not be so. Some national health services are plagued by extravagant waste in the purchase and dispensing of medicines, whereas the wide range of drugs in the formularies from one national plan or group insurance hospital demonstrated that the search for only necessary and efficacious medicines is by no means universal.

What about manufacturers? Here at least one relies on the simple marketplace where profit motives rule. Yet genuine scientific and humanitarian concern is to be found among physicians, researchers and others in the pharmaceutical industry, just as venal motives are not unknown among those working with and for the sick in ostensibly non-profit-making institutions.

The foregoing observations are intended only to keep us mindful of the diversity existing within interest groups as well as among them. Under conditions of such diversity, supplemented by the very powerful health matters at stake, and the immense opportunities for profit – or for purchasers, of loss – one can understand the continuing battles which characterise institutional and sometimes personal interactions in seeking to develop and apply sensible policies and practices for providing consumers with medicines.

However, where the profit motive is absent, inertia may prevail so that effective new medicines never reach the doctor or patient. In the USSR, for example, research institutes have no means or incentives to encourage the manufacture of their discoveries, and manufacturing plants no incentive to incur the costs of installing new equipment and techniques (Binyon, 1979).

Examined as institutions, all of the protagonists in the drama – from doctors to consumers – have each one or more national associations which can promote or defend their interests, *vis-à-vis* one another and the state itself. International associations do, however, appear weak – whether these be voluntary (World Medical Association, International Organisation of Consumer Unions) or are officially chartered, as in the WHO or the UN Narcotics Division. Against these, the economic strength and flexibility of multinational pharmaceutical companies looms large enough to enable one to say that if there are significant adversaries to such corporate interests, these are either governments acting to control corporate activities, or professionals and consumers themselves, acting, in democracies, through their representatives, – and able to act in association and individually in their own best interests because they are well-informed and have arrived at rational positions with respect either to social policies regarding drugs or to their individual conduct in advising on or using medicines.

It is in the service of these latter goals that we would see the utility of this volume. We also hope, as an international group ourselves, to encourage the strengthening of international bodies concerned with the development of drug information and policies, and with their benevolent implementation.

References

Anon. (1976). Distinctions with little difference: pseudo-competition in the pharmaceutical industry. *Drug Ther. Bull. 14*, 53-4

Binyon, M. (1979). Soviet drug industry seeks a cure for its ills. *The Times*, 13 December 1979

Dukes, M.N.G. and Lunde, I. (1979). Measuring the effects of drug control – an emerging challenge. *Pharm. J. 17*, Nov., 511-3

Dunnell, K. and Cartwright, A. (1972). *Medicine Takers, Prescribers and Hoarders*, London, Routledge & Kegan Paul

Haslemere Group (1976). *Who Needs the Drug Companies?* London, Haslemere

Hemminki, E. and Personen, T. (1977). The function of drug company representatives. *Scand. J. Soc. Med. 5*, 105-114

Levinson, C. (1974). *The Multinational Pharmaceutical Industry*, Geneva, International Federation of Chemical and General Workers

McKeown, T. (1979). *The Role of Medicine*, Oxford, Blackwell

Parish, P. (1979). *Medicines: a Guide for Everybody* (2nd edn.), London, Penguin

Pradal, H. (1974). *Guide des médicaments les plus courants* (3rd edn.), Paris, Editions du Seuil

Stimson, G. (1974). Obeying doctor's orders: a view from the other side. *Soc. Sci. Med. 8*, 97-104

UNCTAD (United Nations Conference on Trade and Development) (1975). Major issues in transfer of technology to developing countries: a case study of the pharmaceutical industry. Geneva, UNCTAD, Paper No. TD/B/C.6/4

WHO (World Health Organisation) (1979). The selection of essential drugs. 2nd Report, *Tech. Rep. Ser. 641*

2 THE USE OF MEDICINES FOR ILLNESS

Andrew Herxheimer and Gerry V. Stimson

The ways in which we use medicines are linked to our perceptions of disease. When we attempt to categorise the uses of medicines we must consider the particular belief system which that categorisation implies. This is in part because the uses of medicines are not determined solely by their chemical nature and in part because of the power of ideas in shaping and structuring the world of ill-health. In other words, people assign meanings to drugs and medicines, and these meanings often differ between different groups both within and between cultures.

Western 'scientific' medicine is only one of these belief systems but it is the 'official' or dominant one in much of the world. Many other beliefs must be considered, including of course those of the users of medicines. Western medicine has not always prevailed against other beliefs. This is obvious from the problems of practising Western medicine in cultures with a different tradition, but such divergences occur even within Western societies between 'official' medicine and various other groups in the population. We must therefore examine the use of medicines not only from the viewpoint of official medicine, but also from the points of view of different groups of medicine users.

The Medical Use of Medicines

It is relatively easy to classify the medical uses of medicines because these have grown up with the development of scientific medicine. From this point of view the medical uses of medicines are mostly related to the management of disease. Medicines are used in the prevention of many conditions, and they can aid diagnosis, apart from their well-recognised roles of curing and alleviating disease, and of relieving symptoms. Some of these different uses may overlap and may not be distinguished from one another. This can lead to wrong expectations from the use of medicines, and to wrong use, and it is therefore worth considering the different types of use in some detail.

Prevention of Disease (Prophylaxis)

The best known example is the prevention of infectious diseases.

Immunisation with vaccines, or the use of antimicrobial drugs can prevent many infectious diseases and some dangerous infections that can complicate surgical operations. Likewise disinfectant applications to wounds may prevent their infection.

Nutritional deficiency can be prevented by giving supplements to the diet, though these can perhaps be regarded as food rather than as medicines. Examples are the use of folic acid and iron supplements in pregnancy.

Another type of preventive medication is the use of heparin in surgical patients to prevent venous thrombosis (formation of clots in the veins) and embolism. Recently other drugs such as aspirin and sulfapyrazone which reduce the aggregation of blood platelets (thrombocytes) have been used to prevent myocardial infarction or stroke (cerebral infarction) in people at special risk of these.

The essential feature of prophylactic medication is that it is given to people who are judged to be at risk of developing a disease or condition that they can be protected against. Ideally the prophylactic medication must protect the individual throughout the period of risk, which may range from less than one day to many years. For example, an air traveller who touches down briefly at an airport in a malarious region needs protection only for that day (though the drugs now used have to be taken for the ensuing 3 weeks), whereas someone living there will need it continually. Any individual who has had rheumatic fever probably needs continuous protection against streptococcal infection for many years. Ideally, any prophylactic method should carry negligible risks of its own.

In practice most methods involve some risk, but this is usually extremely small in comparison with the risk of developing the condition they are given to prevent. However, when the disease in question is very rare, or virtually extinct, as smallpox is now, the likelihood of getting it becomes so remote that the risk of serious harm resulting from the vaccine is not very different. This emphasises the point that prophylaxis is worth using only when the balance of risks offers the individual a clear advantage.

Contraception is a special and very important example of prophylaxis that differs from the others mentioned. Here what is prevented is not a disease but a normal condition, pregnancy. As long as pregnancy is not desired, every act of intercourse must be protected. But as soon as the couple want a child the contraceptive effect must be quickly and completely reversible. This is always the case with a short-acting contraceptive such as a mechanical or spermicidal barrier, but not always with a long-acting one. It is worth noting that a contraceptive pill is not necessarily short-acting just because it has to be taken every day: especially after it has been taken for some months the effects may take some time to reverse. It is necessary to take it daily because it would otherwise be unreliable; a partial reversal of the contraceptive effect would occur rapidly in some women.

Hormonal contraceptives alter various bodily functions: an oestrogen/progestogen pill, for example, acts on the hypothalamus and pituitary gland to inhibit ovulation and damps down the cyclical growth of the lining of the womb, so incidentally reducing the menstrual flow. Since the pill is used to maintain these altered physiological conditions, which make pregnancy very unlikely, it can equally well be categorised as a form of maintenance therapy (see below).

Diagnostic Uses

Some drugs are used specifically to help in the diagnosis of disease, mostly as essential or important tools in the investigation of the function of various organs. The best-known group of such drugs are the radiological contrast media, which enable most internal organs to be examined by X-rays. An example is barium sulphate, which is completely insoluble and therefore devoid of any pharmacological action. It is used to outline the oesophagus, stomach and small and large intestines, and to show up their movements on the X-ray screen. Other contrast media which are excreted in the bile and concentrated in the gall-bladder, or concentrated by the kidney and excreted in the urine, are used to examine these organs and to test their function. These drugs are pharmacologically active and have various toxic effects.

Substances with short-lived radioactivity, e.g. compounds of the artificial element technetium, are used for 'scanning' various organs, such as the liver, bones, kidney and brain. The substance is injected into a vein, and is then taken up in various tissues where the radioactivity can be detected with external counters and mapped to show the pattern of uptake, which is often altered by disease.

Specific drugs are also used to stimulate secretion of acid by the stomach (pentagastrin), to stimulate the activity of various glands, and to test other functions.

A special dye, fluorescein, is put in eyedrops which stains any part of the cornea that is damaged. This is a simple way of detecting corneal injuries.

Many sedatives, general anaesthetics and local anaesthetics are used as part of a variety of diagnostic procedures. It would, for example, be very difficult or impossible to perform a bronchoscopy without some sedation and local anaesthesia. But in practice such uses cannot be distinguished from the use of these drugs in 'therapeutic' surgery. This example shows how the same drugs can make important (though not central) contributions to quite different medical procedures.

In a few conditions the patient's symptoms and signs are so rapidly and dramatically impaired by a drug that this is used as a diagnostic test. For example, the muscle weakness of myasthenia gravis is relieved in this way by injection of a short-acting anticholinesterase drug, edrophonium (Tensilon), and the coma of overdosage with morphine or another opiate is reversed by an injection of naloxone. Such diagnostic uses border on the therapeutic use of drugs.

Cure

Medicines cure illness much less commonly than many people believe, if cure is defined as the restoration of health. The main types of medicines which can do this are antimicrobial and antiparasitic drugs, anti-cancer drugs, and antidotes to poisons. It is easy to see how a drug which attacks a microbe can enable the patient's own defences to rid the body of the infection, and similarly with parasites and cancer cells. With an antidote to a poison, the process is somewhat different. An antidote may work by inactivating the poison or by accelerating its removal from the body. Or it may antagonise the poison at its site of action: it may either block its access to the point of action or it may have an opposing effect. Preferably the effect of an antidote should last as long or longer than the effect of the poison, otherwise any improvement in the patient will be only transient, so that repeated doses of the antidote have to be given. This is the case when naloxone is used to treat morphine poisoning.

Drugs can also be curative in some other circumstances. For example, a small kidney stone may lodge in the ureter and cause ureteric colic, that is the intense painful spasm of the muscle of the ureter. A drug given to relax this muscle may allow the stone to move down, and to be passed in the urine, and has then produced a cure. But if other stones were present in the kidney and similar episodes were to recur, it would be debatable whether the termination of a single episode would constitute a cure.

Often a medicine can only lead to a cure when its use is accompanied by a change in faulty habits. For example, in chronic constipation laxatives will give some relief, but the patient's diet and bowel habits must be improved by re-education to a point where medication is no longer needed. Such a cure is only in part due to the medicine, in as much as it has facilitated this re-education.

This illustrates the general point that often several factors contribute to recovery from an illness, and that it may be impossible to assess their relative importance. If medicine or surgery is predominantly responsible, the 'cure' tends to be attributed to it; if the patient's own defences and psychic resources seem to deserve the credit, we may say that the patient has shaken off or overcome the illness. If the illness ordinarily tends to recovery, we regard this as 'spontaneous' and give the credit to nature.

Maintenance Therapy

In health many different biochemical and physiological mechanisms control the functioning of the organs and systems of the body. When in disease one of these regulatory mechanisms ceases to work effectively, long-term use of a medicine can often help to restore the function. There are three main types of such maintenance therapy: the replacement of some essential substance that the body lacks, the takeover by drugs of a failing physiological control system, and the suppression of disease activity.

Replacement Therapy. This is required in nutritional deficiencies, especially vitamin deficiencies, and endocrine deficiencies. 'Replacement' includes not only administration of a substance in amounts that were previously present, but also the provision of additional quantities required because the need for the substance has increased. It thus applies to iron-deficiency anaemia when this is due to a subnormal intake of iron in the diet, or to increased loss of iron from the body, e.g. from blood loss, or in pregnancy from transfer to the fetus. If a deficiency is only temporary, then the patient could be regarded as 'cured' when it has been made good. This would be the case in an otherwise well person who has suffered acute water and salt depletion in a hot, dry climate, who would recover rapidly after replacement of the lost salt and water. The intake of salt and water must then, however, continue at a level which will balance the amounts lost in the sweat, etc. This could be regarded as continued maintenance therapy, but if the individual manages it alone it makes better sense to consider it a part of normal life.

A less obvious kind of nutritional replacement is needed in people who are made ill by some usually harmless constituent of food. Most patients with coeliac disease are allergic to gluten, a protein component of wheat and other grains. They must therefore avoid all bread, cakes and other food made with gluten-containing flour, but they may of course eat anything made from gluten-free flour. A gluten-free diet replaces the normal diet in such patients; it could be regarded as 'negative replacement' therapy, since a noxious substance is removed from the diet. But one could also argue that it was a form of prophylactic treatment, since emergence of the disease is prevented.

Endocrine deficiencies can usually be made good by administering the missing hormone either by mouth (e.g. thyroid hormone) or by injection (e.g. insulin). While it is relatively simple to provide the replacement in the appropriate amounts, it may be difficult or impossible to give it just at those times when the body needs it. The flexible response of many endocrine glands can meet the body's demands for the hormone which may change from hour to hour. Conscious administration of a hormone can never attain such close matching of supply to demand. In this sense a perfect replacement of endocrine deficiency could only be achieved if the defective gland were replaced by a well-functioning graft.

Take-over of Homeostatic Control. When the body's regulatory mechanisms do not suffice to restore normal function, drugs can sometimes help. For example, in hypertension the mechanisms controlling the blood pressure are set to keep it at a higher level than normal. Drugs can be used to lower the blood pressure towards normal, and this will prevent some of the harmful consequences of the raised blood pressure, but their effect only continues while the drug is present in the body. Unless the hypertension is temporary, use of the drug must therefore be continued for many years.

Another example of failure in the homeostatic control system is the accumulation of excessive fluid in the circulation and the tissues (dropsy) when the heart begins to fail. Drugs which increase the force of contraction of the heart, so that it pumps round the blood more efficiently, can reduce this accumulation of fluid, and so can diuretics which act on the kidney to increase the excretion of water and salts into the urine. In myasthenia gravis the muscles are weak because the nerves supplying them release too little acetylcholine, the substance that stimulates the muscle fibre to contract. Muscle power can be restored by giving a drug (e.g. neostigmine) which delays the destruction of acetylcholine, and so increases its concentration at the point where it acts on the muscle fibre.

In asthma the airways are narrowed by bronchial muscle spasm and obstructed by sticky secretions. The physiological mechanisms for dilating the bronchi and getting rid of the excessive secretions are inadequate, and can be reinforced by drugs which relax the bronchial muscle or which make the secretions thinner and more easily coughed up. Again, treatment with such drugs is needed for as long as the bronchial obstruction persists, but the intensity of the treatment must correspond to the intensity of the need for it. Because breathlessness, cough and wheezing are relieved by this type of treatment, it can equally be regarded as symptomatic therapy (see below).

Suppression of the Disease Process. Some drugs can interfere with the expression of the disease process, so that its manifestations are subdued or abolished. For example, one of the actions of corticosteroid drugs is to suppress inflammatory reactions, and to inhibit various immune responses. Rheumatoid arthritis, and various allergic diseases are suppressed in this way, but only temporarily, while the drug is being used. If a disease is self-limited then it can be alleviated or suppressed until spontaneous recovery occurs. This is the case in hay fever, where the condition lasts only for 6 to 8 weeks, usually in May and June. Immunosuppressive therapy is used to prevent the rejection of transplanted organs by the host, e.g. a transplanted kidney. This can also be regarded as prophylactic treatment.

Symptomatic Treatment

This treatment is used to relieve or prevent a symptom, such as pain, fever, cough, nausea, itching. The term is not used for treatment that affects the disease which is causing the symptom. It does not necessarily do anything to correct the disturbance associated with the symptom. It is not practicable to use a drug to prevent a symptom unless its occurrence can be reliably predicted. Examples are the use of glyceryl trinitrate before exercise to prevent angina pectoris, of an antacid an hour after a meal to prevent the pain associated with duodenal ulcer, or of a sleeping pill to prevent insomnia.

In some circumstances a drug used to relieve a symptom may actually exacerbate or worsen the condition causing the symptom. For example, morphine may, by an action on the brain, relieve the severe pain caused by spasm of the intestine or the bile-duct, while at the same time making the spasm more intense. Aspirin, paracetamol and similar drugs are often used to reduce fever, but in many infections fever probably contributes to the defence against the infectious agent. Alcohol is a notorious example. It will quickly comfort the chilled traveller with a warm glow, but unless the body is kept warm it also greatly increases heat loss from the skin and consequently the risk of serious hypothermia.

Symptomatic remedies usually have a relatively brief action; their effect does not persist after the drug has been eliminated from the body. The patient knows better than anyone else whether and to what extent the treatment relieves symptoms and is also most likely to know how inconvenient the treatment is. It is therefore appropriate for the patient to control symptomatic treatment if this can be managed. Most drugs used in self-medication are symptomatic remedies.

Compliance

Much of what we know about the way in which people use prescribed medicines comes, in a rather negative fashion, from studies which have tried to find reasons for patients' non-compliance with doctors' instructions. These drug-use studies have generally used some version of the following method: a known quantity of medicine is prescribed to a particular patient sample and some technique is then used to monitor patients' use of this medicine — how much is taken, how often, and when. Techniques might be urine testing, questioning, or counting how much remains. The amount unused in the time period is compared to the amount that should have been used, to derive some measure of 'non-compliance'.

The above studies find that a substantial proportion of patients do not follow instructions; the percentage defaulting ranges from 19-72 per cent in outpatient and general practice contexts (Stimson, 1974). The majority of studies put the percentage of patients defaulting at 30 or more. These studies have been conducted on a variety of different people such as children, the elderly chronic sick, TB patients, pregnant women, and those discharged from psychiatric hospitals. They have been given a variety of different drugs — penicillin, tranquillisers, iron, antibiotics and TB drugs. Studies of compliance have been comprehensively and critically reviewed by Sackett and Haynes (1976).

Most investigators have been unsuccessful in identifying a particular type of patient who 'defaults', except in the clear case of people who have memory problems — such as the old. The therapeutic regimen is important — where more than one drug is prescribed or a drug has inconvenient side effects the medication is less likely to be used as directed. But beyond these rather obvious factors it seems that 'non-compliance' is explicable less in terms of types of people and in the technicalities of therapeutic regimens, than in the contexts of patients' beliefs and the nature of the doctor-patient interaction.

Studies which have attempted to link patient beliefs and expectations and doctor-patient interaction have been more successful. For example, Francis, Korsch and Morris (1969) studied outpatient visits to a paediatric department and found that mothers who expected to learn the causation and nature of their child's illness and who failed to do so were less likely to be satisfied and less likely to follow medical advice than any other group of patients. Patients who expected laboratory tests, X-rays or injections and did not receive them were less compliant than the rest of the sample. Other investigators using different approaches have shown that the doctor-patient interaction is crucial for subsequent patient behaviour. Davis (1968) found that patients' failure to comply was associated with a pattern of interaction in the consultation characterised by formality, antagonism, and the mutual withholding of information and expression.

Studies of defaulting seem to suggest that all medication is to some extent self-medication, even if it is not self-prescribed. Except in those rare situations where treatment can be forced on the patient, it is usually the case that medication can take place only at the initiative of or with the consent of the patient. Patients' ideas and attitudes towards medication, expectations of treatment, beliefs about health and illness, experience with the treatment, and advice from friends and relatives are all likely to influence the use of treatments. Many influences have an important bearing on when medical care is sought; such influences also support, antagonise or otherwise modify prescriptions and regimens dispensed by those officially charged with the patients' treatment and care.

The Scientific Ideal and the Practical Reality in Western Medicine

Within the medical profession actual practice may depart from the rational model of use proposed in the official view of the professional élite. Given the variety of specialists and groupings within medicine consensus on practice is unlikely. Indeed, the classic studies of drug innovation show that it takes time for ideas to spread and practices to change (Coleman, 1966), and we find evidence of variability in prescribing practices and changing fashions in prescribing (Parish *et al.*, 1976; Parish, 1975). We also find other 'non-rational practices', for example prescribing determined more by the social acceptability of certain drugs than on pharmacological grounds, non-scientific placebo prescribing (Comaroff, 1976); prescribing to facilitate interaction, for example as a way to end a consultation (Stimson and Webb, 1975); as a response to perceived patient demand (Stimson, 1976); or when doctors are at a loss to know what other action to take (Lennard *et al.*, 1971).

While on the one hand there are pressures towards scientific and rational prescribing, a good case can be made that aspects of the practice of medicine predispose towards some undesirable outcomes. Freidson (1975) argues that there is a 'bias towards illness in everyday practice' and Scheff (1963) that one 'medical decision rule' is that physicians typically assume that, in an uncertain diagnostic situation, it is better to impute disease in the patient than to deny it and risk missing it. It would follow that we could consider such practices as 'unnecessary surgery' and 'overprescribing' as natural consequences of medical practice and not the result of aberrant practice.

The final comment that must be made about the rationalist medical view is that medical practice contains more than the attempt to tackle illness and treat 'justifiable pain'. The intentions of doctors are not always confined to medical treatment to benefit the sick individual. There is a growing critique that medical practice has become involved in social control, that is, to adjust behaviour in the direction of normative expectations. Examples are the use of drugs to control prisoners (*Guardian*, 1976, PROP 1978), to control hyperactive school children (*Drug & Therapeutics Bulletin*, 1977) and as management devices in hospital wards (for example, see the promotional booklet for Valium, Roche Products 1968).

In the area of drug abuse, one of the UK medical responses has been 'competitive prescribing' to lure addicts from the black market. The aim is to control the size and spread of the drug problem. British treatment for drug addicts is a peculiar example of medical practice because some of the doctors actually refer to their work as 'control' and 'containment' (Stimson, 1978). The point about social control is that the doctor is not the agent of the patient but of some third party, and the aim is not primarily the patient's welfare but the welfare of others troubled by the patient.

Since we can so easily find examples within medicine where there is a marked divergence of practice from the official model, it should not surprise us to find that the further we get from the domain of medical influence the more we should expect peoples' views, knowledge, motivation and practices to diverge from medical ones.

Lay Views on the Use of Medicines

A major problem for such a task is the categories we use to interpret patient behaviour. A patient who does not use prescribed drugs as directed by the doctor is called 'non-compliant', but we must entertain the possibility that this 'non-compliance' is a sensible, rational and meaningful response from the point of view of the patient. The categories which are available are often the official categories, and these may distort our understanding of the phenomenon. It is easy to see in the case of illicit drug use how our categories have this distorting effect — our view of heroin use among American servicemen in Vietnam varied according to whether we called it 'abuse', 'recreational use' or 'self-medication'. The categories we use are rarely derived from the experience of the people concerned; and, of course, even the categories we use can change — one has only to look at the changing views about opiates in the last hundred years.

The dominant official medical view is historically linked in the West, with the definition of certain forms of chemical use as illegitimate (Berridge, 1978). This dominant perspective may in turn be linked with the lack of interest in systems of indigenous medicine and self-medication, and accounts for the paucity of research in these areas (Zola, 1976).

We sometimes know more about the meanings of medicine use and lay conceptions of health and illness in exotic cultures and tribal societies. The classic work of Frake (1961) on the diagnosis of disease among the Subanum of Mindanao, Maclean's work on Nigerian medicine (1971) and Schwartz's work on the explanation of the cause of illness and the choice of native or Western curative practices (1969) are the sorts of studies that we need in developed societies.

Unfortunately, we generally know little about the motivation and meanings of peoples' use of drugs. We have various surveys from developed countries of 'who uses what', but these have not been designed to look at the questions we are mainly interested in — why, when and how do people use medicines? Very often we have to use these data to make inferences about beliefs, with the danger that alternative interpretations are possible.

Medication Use and Belief System

Too much emphasis on medications — on the techniques of medical practice — can mislead us over the intention with which medications are used or over the choice of medications. Our primary interest in this book is in medications, but it is difficult to separate medication use from the context or belief system which suggests the correct way to behave in the case of illness. What the Western doctor may see as the correct way may be mystifying to an African and what an African traditional healer sees as the correct way may be equally mystifying to the Western doctor. Western medicine has made its scientific advances by predominantly concerning itself with the somatic causation of disease. In practice, once the doctor has defined the illness according to a particular cluster of signs and symptoms, he can then offer a diagnosis and a prescription. In many cultures this is not sufficient for the patient, nor even the most important aspect. In many cultures the sick person requires an explanation of the particularity of the individual misfortune — answers to the questions: Why me? Why now? Why in this particular way? A quote from Maclean (1971, p. 28) well illustrates this point:

> For the Nigerian who falls ill whilst on a visit to his brother it is not a sufficient explanation to be told that he has an attack of dysentery. He was well enough when he left home, why should he be suddenly incapacitated now, why is no one else affected? The suggestion of a germ in his food will only lead him to demand how it got there, more explicitly *who* put it there. In his own mind he recalls the hesitation with which he had regarded this journey, the reluctance he felt to encounter a stepbrother whose feelings for him had always been uncertain; he broods upon the likelihood that his food was tampered with by his brother's jealous wife. Speculations and suspicions such as these will preoccupy his attention and may subsequently determine the counter-measures which he decides to employ.

It has only been recently recognised that people in developed societies also ask this kind of question. There is a powerful moral aspect to illness, and people seek out the reasons why they are now ill. They may not believe that their food has been tampered with, but illness, and certainly recurrent illness, is often explained in terms of personal moral responsibility. Ironically, with the discovery of the link between life-events and illness (Brown, 1976), the psychosomatic basis of some illnesses, and that infective organisms are often present in the body without illness occurring, Western scientific medicine seems to be coming, slowly, in a full circle to a scientific confirmation of this pre-scientific mode of thinking about illness.

What do People do When They are Ill?

Medicines use must be viewed in the context of action people take when they experience symptoms — in the setting of what social scientists call 'illness behaviour'. Epidemiological studies show that the experience of symptoms is the norm rather than the exception. The findings of the Dunnell and Cartwright (1972) study are typical. They undertook a survey of peoples' use of prescribed and over-the-counter medicines in the United Kingdom. The vast majority of people (83 per cent) rated their health as 'excellent' or 'good' over the previous two weeks. Paradoxically, whilst the majority felt healthy, they were not free from symptoms. Only 9 per cent of the adults said that they did not have any of a checklist of symptoms during the same two weeks. For example, 32 per cent reported coughs, catarrh or phlegm; 38 per cent had had headaches; 6 per cent had palpitations or a thumping heart.

The average number of reported symptoms for the two weeks was 3.9. Taking the family as a survey unit, a US panel study found that on average families were dealing with one illness episode every four days (Knapp and Knapp, 1972). Such studies remind us that illness is very much a feature of everyday life. Ogden Nash says much the same in the introduction to *Family Reunion*: 'The family is a unit composed not only of children, but men, women, the occasional animal — and the common cold' (quoted in Robinson, 1971).

Little of this illness is taken to a doctor. All such studies confirm that the doctor only sees a minute proportion of illness. In the Dunnell and Cartwright study (1972) although 91 per cent of the adults reported symptoms during the two weeks, only 16 per cent had consulted a doctor in that time, and 28 per cent said that they had not consulted their general practitioner at all during the previous 12 months. Horder and Horder (1954) estimated that only a third of illnesses reached a medical agency, but even this must be an over-estimate because more recent work shows, for example, that only one in 184 episodes of headaches was taken to a doctor (Banks *et al.*, 1975).

In a 1949 UK survey Logan and Brook (1957) found that less than one in four of those complaining of illness had seen a doctor about the complaint. The findings from a health survey of a London borough by Wadsworth, Butterfield and Blaney (1971) show that in a community of one thousand people over the age of 16, the vast majority (750-900) have in any given two weeks at least one painful and distressing symptom. Only about 200 would have visited any type of doctor during the same period. Of this 200, about 136 would have visited a general practitioner or been visited by one, 28 would have attended as out-patients at a hospital, and only five would have been in-patients.

The above evidence is a striking confirmation of Davis' point that 'a considerable portion of the individual's health and illness experience takes place in locales and with persons far removed from the guidance and control of institutionalised medical authority – in the home, at work, with kin, friends, neighbours, and others in the person's routine orbit of existence' (1963). Perhaps this point may seem unnecessary to a reader who lives in a society where much indigenous medicine is still the norm and where Western medical facilities are rare: the point is, that Western medicine only every so often rediscovers that it sees merely a small proportion of the illness experienced in any community.

What action do people take when they are ill? The epidemiological studies indicate a high level of medication, particularly self-medication. Given the high level of symptoms, perhaps our main question should not be why people medicate, but why some people do not, for medication is the norm.

In a UK study 55 per cent of the adults had taken some kind of medication in the previous 24 hours, taken an average 2.2 items in a two-week period (Dunnell and Cartwright, 1972). An international study of three towns in the United States, United Kingdom, and Yugoslavia found that respectively 48, 38 and 19 per cent had taken a prescribed or over-the-counter medicine in the last 24 hours (White *et al.*, 1967). A US panel survey found that 95 per cent of households had procured at least one drug in a 30-week period, and on average procured 13.7 (Knapp and Knapp, 1972). In most surveys the use of over-the-counter (non-prescription) drugs exceeds the use of prescription drugs, but the ratio will vary, amongst other things, by the relative prices, the system of medical care, medical beliefs, etc. However, regardless of prescription use, self-medication seems to be the norm; in the Dunnell and Cartwright study 60 per cent of those interviewed used a non-prescribed medication in a 2-week period and Knapp and Knapp (1972) found that non-prescribed drugs were used in 70 per cent of illness incidents.

It is the case then that much illness is not taken to the doctor but self-treated; surveys in developed countries rediscover much of what is taken for granted in underdeveloped ones. 'Indigenous' or folk medicine is practised throughout the world; it is not confined to underdeveloped countries, nor in developed countries can it simply be viewed as a relic of a folk past.

The great variety of national conditions poses a difficulty for such a review as this. Social science surveys are features of a high level of industrial development, and so we tend to know little of medical practices in underdeveloped countries. What we do know is that the consumption of *manufactured* pharmaceuticals increases when there is an increase in the population which is more likely to use medicines – the chronically ill, when there is greater access to care (Rabin and Bush, 1974) and with increasing industrialisation, affluence and technology.

Manufactured pharmaceuticals are expensive. In the UK, the annual per capita expenditure on pharmaceuticals alone in 1971 was in the region of £50 while in Tanzania, per capita expenditure on *all* official health services in 1972 was £1.15 (Gish, 1975) and the expenditure on pharmaceuticals accounted for about 23 per cent of this sum. In the UK in 1969 the amount was £40 (Leeson, 1974), with pharmaceuticals accounting for 10 per cent of this. An anthropologist observed that in one Indian village some families spent *no* money on medical care whatsoever, not even on traditional remedies (Beals, 1976).

In many underdeveloped countries Western medical practitioners are rare. In Nigeria in the 1960s some regions had only one doctor for every 100,000 of the population. It is not surprising then that much health care in non-industrial countries is practised by traditional healers. It has been estimated that there is one traditional healer for every 500 population in Lagos (Maclean, 1971), and one for every 400 in Dar es Salaam, Tanzania (Gish, 1975). The anthropological literature shows that traditional medicine persists. Even so, we must not make the assumption that most illness is taken to a traditional healer. In underdeveloped as in developed societies, self-treatment is the first resort.

Drugs in the Home

In Nigeria, it may be herbal medications or locally made medicines which are used. The Western equivalent of medicinal herbs are manufactured pharmaceuticals. Ninety-nine per cent of households surveyed in a UK study had medicines in the home, with an average of 3.0 prescribed items and 7.3 non-prescribed ones (Dunnell and Cartwright, 1972). A US study found an average 5.3 prescribed and 17.2 non-prescribed items in the home (Knapp and Knapp, 1972). In the UK study 85 per cent of households had analgesics, 43 per cent laxatives, 48 per cent skincreams, 20 per cent sedatives, sleeping tablets or tranquillisers and 29 per cent had vitamins or iron tablets. People of higher social class had more medicines, but this may reflect different patterns of purchasing rather than of consumption. The higher use rates for the US compared to other countries (White *et al.*, 1967) might also be a function of income.

Few of the above studies give any idea of why people keep medicines in the home. Dunnell and Cartwright speculate that many prescribed medicines are kept because people forget to throw them away when the illness has passed. That people might not intend to use them again is indicated by the willingness with which they are given up to drug collection programmes (Nicholson, 1967). Half of the unused antibiotics in the home had first been obtained more than a year ago. Other types of medicines are kept for when they might be needed — 40 per cent of analgesics in the home had not been used in the last month.

Patterns of Medication

We can infer something of health beliefs in data from medication use studies which show that in developed countries the most common self-prescribed drugs are analgesics, digestives and laxatives, preparations for coughs and colds and vitamins: for example, in the UK these groups account for two-thirds of sales on non-prescribed medicines (Price Commission, 1978; Blum *et al.*, 1969). These products are advertised by manufacturers and the extent of their use indicates both health beliefs and advertising practices.

In developed countries it is probably unrealistic to conceive of a realm of 'traditional' beliefs independent of such influences as advertising, and it would be important to analyse the relationship between the two. We should not think of the influence as one way — that advertising directly moulds health beliefs — for advertising is designed to both reflect and to reinforce pre-existing ideas. For example, advertisers take traditional beliefs about ill-health, such as the role of the wife/mother as family nurse, use these beliefs in advertising imagery, and in turn reinforce such beliefs.

In the UK people are more likely to medicate headaches, constipation, sore throats, indigestion and ulcers, than to medicate breathlessness, dizziness or varicose veins (Dunnell and Cartwright, 1972; Jeffreys *et al.*, 1960). Approaching the question from another direction, Banks *et al.* (1975) related the experience of symptoms to consultation behaviour. A prospective diary study of women in the UK found that there were different rates of consultation for different symptoms. Only one episode of headaches in 184 led a patient to consult, but 1 in 18 episodes of sore throats led to a consultation. Symptoms least likely to lead to a consultation (and thus possibly more likely to be self-treated) were changes in energy, headache, disturbance of gastric function, backache, pain in lower limb and emotional symptoms — all these led to consultations at about one in 50 or fewer episodes.

Do Some People Medicate More than Others?

It is difficult to know what characteristics we should look for. At the hypochondriacal fringe there may be clear characteristics, but most investigators have had little success in isolating characteristics of different types of users — admittedly most of them have confined themselves to relatively simple demographic indicators. Thus from one study: 'our attempt to identify medicine takers by such characteristics as age, sex and social class has been in many ways abortive. Apparent associations between age, social class and medication can be explained simply in terms of the amount of perceived ill health' (Dunnell and Cartwright, 1972). And from another study: 'our attempts to find any distinguishing characteristics of the adult men and women who took self-prescribed medicines as compared with those who did not were singularly unsuccessful' (Jeffreys *et al.*, 1960). Blum *et al.* (1969) did find differences, but possibly because they included extremes of medication use from normal use of alcohol up to use of illicit drugs.

Similar negative findings come from studies which have looked at the related question of the characteristics of people who frequently consult the doctor or that special group of people who rarely consult at all. In a study of 10-year non-attenders of a middle-class general practice in a suburb of London, 3 per cent had not attended in this time. There was little difference between them and the attenders except that they tended to see themselves as healthy, and tended to use fewer self-prescribed medicines, but only to the extent that 25 per cent did not self-medicate (Kessel and Shepherd, 1965).

The lack of success in distinguishing people who medicate in different ways is probably due to the fact that the important belief systems and illness practices are not in any clear way linked to simple demographic characteristics.

Reasons for Self-medication

We are dwelling on self-medication because it is statistically more common than prescribed medication and because it helps us to focus on the main context of health and illness — peoples' everyday lives. It is clear from studies of the 'process of becoming ill' and of peoples' help-seeking behaviour, that consulting a doctor is not the commonest sort of action in the case of illness. People seek a whole range of lay and other advice-givers when they are ill. McKinlay (1970) found that women who had a readily available network of friends and kin were less likely to seek professional advice. Zola (1973) found that usually people accommodated to symptoms, and that it was often only after changes in a person's family and social situation occurred that a consultation followed.

The first source of advice that is usually taken is likely to be lay advice. Freidson (1961) likens lay advice to a 'lay referral system' along which a person is referred until there is no more lay advice and the next course of action is to consult a doctor. Self-medication then is one of a number of alternatives available when illness is experienced. In fact we must not overlook *no* action as an alternative — in one study 47 per cent of symptoms were not medicated (Dunnell and Cartwright, 1972).

From the published studies we can infer when and why self-medication might be used. The evidence suggests several different reasons: firstly, when the illness experienced is not of the sort that is usually taken to the doctor, because it is of a trivial and easily self-treatable nature — such as headaches, indigestion, and first-aid for cuts and abrasions; secondly, when the doctor is not available because he is not easily accessible (in some parts of some countries there might be no doctor available), or because of financial or other barriers to consultations; thirdly, self-medication may be used as a stop-gap to relieve symptoms until medical advice can be sought; and fourthly, when illness is seen to be not of the sort that doctors can do much about. Many of the advertised remedies are for symptoms which are generally self-limiting, or for which medical intervention is of little help – the common cold, arthritis, or indigestion. Fifthly, when 'official' medicine has proved to be ineffective, people may resort to self-medication.

Several commentators have sought to establish whether self-medication is a supplement to or alternative to prescribed medication. Jefferys found that on the whole it was not an alternative – the majority of those who took prescribed medicines supplemented them with self-prescribed medicines (Jefferys *et al.*, 1960). This link has been reversed to some extent in other studies (Dunnell and Cartwright, 1972). We might also ask the question whether self-medication is used as a first resort, or as a last resort after prescribed medication has failed. It is unlikely that we shall find an easy 'either/or' answer. People have a range of resources in illness. Different medical systems can exist side by side, and not only in underdeveloped countries, in part because they address themselves to different aspects of the disease situation (Leeson, 1974).

What can we infer about intentions? As in official medicine, we can identify uses of medicines similar to those which have been outlined earlier in this chapter. Medicines may be used for *prevention*; in one study 30 per cent of the adults who had no illness or symptoms were taking medicines (Jefferys *et al.*, 1960). Medicine-taking can be *prophylactic* – possibly much laxative use falls into this category. Antiseptics and gargles are taken to reduce the risk of infection. *Symptomatic* treatment is probably the biggest single reason and accounts for the widespread use of aspirins and analgesics. *Replacement* treatment may be a perceived use of vitamins and food supplements. Undoubtedly, many people think of some self-treatments as *cures*, and sometimes even the medical profession may concede some validity in such claims – the medical dispute about the benefits of vitamin C for the common cold is a case in point. To this list we should add *health promotion*, which is slightly different from the prevention of ill health. This we would see as the aim of the natural health movement (Roth, 1978), the use of vitamins and ginseng, and attention to dietary practice. Vitamins are taken by 6 per cent of the UK population (Dunnell and Cartwright, 1972).

The same classes of drugs can be put into different categories according to the inferred intention of their use. Furthermore, people (like doctors) can accept non-rational uses of medicines to achieve other ends – like giving a sick child a medicine in the knowledge that it does not have any effects on the illness, but to convince the child that he or she is being helped. Medicines can be used as placebos or devices to encourage optimism and speed recovery.

There are certainly some patterns of medication where drug use has changed from an isolated event used with some specific intention, into an everyday routine or perhaps compulsion. The use of aspirin or other analgesics is a good example. They are the most common self-prescribed medications, used on a daily basis by 2.8 per cent of the UK population (National Opinions Poll, 1970). Excessive use of analgesics is associated with potential harm. This has been well documented by Murray *et al.* (1970) and Murray (1973a) who found that 51 patients with analgesic nephropathy (1973b) had an average intake of 6 doses of an analgesic daily for 20 years. Patients who were daily users were more likely to give a family history of analgesic abuse and alcoholism and were more likely to have attempted suicide, seen a psychiatrist or be prescribed psychotropic drugs. This group of patients is interesting because they saw themselves that their analgesic use had become a habit, and because the majority of users reported that they took analgesics primarily for their mood-altering quality. Only two had a clear organic reason for taking them.

One final point should be made about intentions – we cannot ignore self-medication and its connection with suicide, euthanasia and self-poisoning. In London, one adult in every 230 takes an overdose, deliberate or otherwise, during the course of one year. In cases of deliberate self-poisoning (about 60 per cent of poisoning episodes, but of course there is difficulty in classification) psychoactive drugs of some sort were used in 71 per cent of incidents, and analgesics in 29 per cent (there is some overlap due to more than one drug being taken) (Ghodse, 1976, 1977).

Sources of Information About Health, Illness and Treatment

Few would deny the power of the medical profession in developed countries to pronounce on the nature of illness and its treatment. This has been the substance of extensive analysis and criticisms (see e.g. Freidson, 1975; Illich, 1975). Concomitant with the rise of an organised medical profession, many traditional beliefs have been rejected as irrational. In Europe and North America female traditional healers were suppressed, their remedies became old wives' tales, and the practice of medicine became the province of men (Ehrenreich and English, 1972). In colonial and neocolonial societies traditional medicine was rejected by Western doctors as 'the mumbo-jumbo of witch doctors'. In only a few parts of the world has there been a conscious effort to retain the best of traditional medicine. This has happened in China, and the *Barefoot Doctors' Manual* lists for each disease the traditional Chinese treatments as well as the modern Western medical ones (and, it is interesting to note, treatment descriptions are preceded by a section on prevention for each disease) (Fogarty International Center, 1974).

In developed countries, indigenous medicine has not been entirely lost. In the West in recent years, there has been a revival of the ethno-pharmacopoeic tradition — not through word of mouth or the passing of the tradition from generation to generation as much as through books. Books such as Culpeper's on herbal treatments are frequently re-published. One English book, Potter's *New Cyclopaedia of Botanical Drugs and Preparations* had seen 10 editions since it was first published in 1907 (Wren, 1971). Books on herbal treatments have the express intention of self-treatment, as is clearly shown in the title of the *Complete Herbalist: or, The People their own Physician* (Brown, 1916). The cover of Jarvis' book on folk medicine mentions the cure and treatment of the common cold, hay fever, arthritis, kidney trouble, digestive disorders, overweight, high blood pressure and chronic fatigue — some of which have no official effective treatments. It has run to 14 editions since 1971 (Jarvis, 1971).

The rationalist side of the self-treatment movement has aimed to bring people more knowledge about: drug treatment (Pradal, 1974; Parish, 1976); self-help (Robinson and Henry, 1977) and self-examination (MacKeith, 1976); about occupational and chemical hazards to health (Kinnersly, 1973); or simply practical advice on medicine in the absence of doctors, as in the *Sierra Club Wilderness Handbook* (Brower, 1971). The ideology and practice of self-help, self-treatment and self-care is part of a 1970s reaction against professionalism in industrial countries, what one commentator has referred to as 'deprofessionalisation' and the 'revolt of the client' (Haug, 1975). However, it is difficult to estimate the impact of these revived approaches as alternatives to or modifiers of organised medicine.

Even in literate societies few people read books and although we take popular publications as indicative of changing sentiments, we would be unwise to overestimate their impact. The media are more accessible sources of information on health and illness. A glance at any newspaper or magazine will show that a considerable proportion is given over to news and articles on medicine and illness (Best *et al.*, 1978), romance stories about doctors and nurses, stories of peoples' triumphs over severe illness, advertisements for non-prescribed medicines, and advice columns. One popular US columnist receives over 1,000 letters a day and has an estimated readership of 54 million. Seventy-two per cent of letters sent to one columnist were from women, and 77 per cent sought advice or a solution to a problem (Dibner, 1974). In recent years radio chat shows and 'phone-in' programmes have increasingly covered medical and emotional problems.

As we have seen already, relatives and friends continue to be a major source of advice in illness and a main source of recommendation for the use of self-prescribed medicines (McKinlay, 1970; Dunnell and Cartwright, 1972).

Conclusions

We are only beginning to discover peoples' belief systems about the use of medicines. Such has been the dominance of the official medical view that indigenous medical practices are seldom researched, are dismissed as of little importance, or only deemed worthy of investigation when they cause problems for professionals, such as patient non-compliance. We can only briefly touch on these belief systems because of the great variety throughout the world, and because we often have to make inferences from data not designed to examine them. The main conclusions of this review are that, despite the rise of modern medicine, it would be unwise to view people as relying solely on official medicine for their remedies and treatment. The bulk of treatment of everyday illness is not taken to doctors; self-treatment is the norm. Secondly, even when it is taken to doctors, people tend to remain in control and do not hand all decision-making over to the doctor. They are best viewed not as passive, obedient recipients of medical care, but as actively involved in their own illness and its treatment.

References

ABPI (Association of the British Pharmaceutical Industry) (1977). *Annual Report*, 1976-7

Banks, M.H., Beresford, S.A.A., Morrell, D.C., Wallen, J.J. and Watkins, C.J. (1975). Factors influencing the demand for primary medical care in women aged twenty to forty-four: a preliminary report. *Int. J. Epidemiology 4*,

3, 189-95

Beals, A.R. (1976). Strategies of resort to curers in South India. In *Asian Medical Systems*, Leslie, C. (ed.), Berkeley, University of California Press

Berridge, V. (1978). Professionalization and narcotics: the medical and pharmaceutical profession and British narcotic use 1868-1926. *Psychological Medicine 8*

Best, G., Dennis, J. and Draper, P. (1978). *Health, the Mass Media, and the National Health Service*, London, Unit for the Study of Health Policy, Guy's Hospital

Blum, R.H., Braunstein, L. and Stone, A. (1969). Normal drug use: an exploratory study of patterns and correlates. In Cole, J.O. and Wittenborn, J.R. (eds.), *Drug Abuse*, Springfield, Illinois, Charles C. Thomas, 59-92

Brower, D. (ed.) (1971). *Sierra Club Wilderness Handbook*, New York, Ballantine

Brown, G.W. (1976). Social causes of disease. Chapter 9 in *Introduction to Medical Sociology*, Tuckett, D. (ed.), London, Tavistock Publications

Brown, O.P. (1916). *The Complete Herbalist: or, The People their own Physicians*, Huddersfield, O.P. Brown Ltd

Coleman, J., Katz, E. and Menzel, M. (1966). *Medical Innovation*, New York, Bobbs-Merrill

Comaroff, J. (1976). A bitter pill to swallow: placebo therapy in general practice. *Sociological Review 24*, 1, 79-96

Davis, F. (1963). *Passage Through Crisis*, Indianapolis, Bobbs-Merrill

Davis, M.S. (1968). Variations in patients' compliance with doctors' advice: an empirical analysis of patterns of communication. *American J. Publ. Health 56*, 274-88

Dibner, S.S. (1974). Newspaper advice columns as a mental health resource. *Community Mental Health Journal 10*, 2, 147-155

Drug and Therapeutics Bulletin (1977). Stimulant drugs for hyperactive children. *15*, 22-4

Dunnell, K. and Cartwright, A. (1972). *Medicine Takers, Hoarders and Prescribers*, London, Routledge and Kegan Paul

Ehrenreich, B. and English, D. (1972). *Witches, Midwives and Nurses: a History of Women Healers*, (2nd edn.), Old Westbury, NY, The Feminist Press

Fogarty International Centre (1974). *A Barefoot Doctor's Manual*, US Dept. of Health Education and Welfare, Publication NIH 75-695

Frake, C.O. (1961). The diagnosis of disease among the Subanum of Mindanao. *Amer. Anthrop. 63*, 113-32

Francis, V., Korsch, B.M. and Morris, M.J. (1969). Gaps in doctor-patient communication. *New England Journal of Medicine 280*, 10, 535-40

Freidson, E. (1961). *Patients' Views of Medical Practice*, New York, Russell Sage Foundation

Freidson, E. (1975). *Profession of Medicine*, New York, Dodd-Mead

Ghodse, A.H. (1976). Drug problems dealt with by 62 London casualty departments. *Brit. J. Prev. Soc. Med. 30*, 4, 251-6

Ghodse, A.H. (1977). Deliberate self-poisoning: a study in London casualty departments. *British Medical Journal 1*, 805-8

Gish, O. (1975). *Planning the Health Service: The Tanzanian Experience*, London, Croom Helm

Guardian (newspaper) (1 October 1976)

Haug, M. (1975). Deprofessionalisation – an alternate hypothesis for the future. *Sociological Review Monography 20*, 195-211

Horder, J. and Horder, E. (1954). Illness in general practice. *Practitioner 173*, 177-87

Illich, I. (1975). *Medical Nemesis: The Expropriation of Health*, London, Calder & Boyars

Jarvis, D.C. (1971). *Folk Medicine*, London, Pan Books

Jefferys, M., Brotherston, J.H.F. and Cartwright, A. (1960). Consumption of medicines on a working-class housing estate. *Brit. J. Prev. Soc. Med. 14*, 64-76

Kessel, N. and Shepherd, M. (1965). The health and attitudes of people who seldom consult a doctor. *Medical Care 3*, 1, 6-10

Kinnersly, P. (1973). *The Hazards of Work: How to Fight Them*, London, Pluto Press

Knapp, D.A. and Knapp, D.E. (1972). Decision making and self-medication: preliminary findings. *Amer. J. Hosp. Pharmacy. 29*, 1004-12

Leeson, J. (1974). Social science and health policy in preindustrial society. *Int. J. Health Serv. 4*, 3, 429-40

Lennard, H., Epstein, L.J., Bernstein, A. and Ransom, D.C. (1971). *Mystification and Drug Misuse*, San Francisco, Jossey-Bass

Logan, W.P.D. and Brooke, E.M. (1957). The Survey of Sickness, 1954-1952. *Studies on Medical and Population Subjects 12* HMSO

MacKeith, N. (1976). *Women's Health Handbook*, Leeds, Virago

Maclean, U. (1971). *Magical Medicine: A Nigerian Case Study*, London, Allen Lane

McKinlay, J.S. (1970). Social networks, lay consultation and help-seeking behaviour. *Social Forces 51*, 275-92

Murray, R.M., Timbury, G.C. and Linton, A.L. (1970). Analgesic abuse in psychiatric patients. *Lancet* 1303-5

Murray, R.M. (1973a). Patterns of analgesic use and abuse in medical patients. *The Practitioner 211*, 639

Murray, R.M. (1973b). Dependence on analgesics in analgesic nephropathy. *Brit. J. Addict. 68*, 265-72

National Opinions Poll, (1970). Survey on powders and tablets. NOP 14256

Nicholson, W.A. (1967). Collection of unwanted drugs from private homes. *Brit. Med. J. 3*, 730-1

Parish, P. (1975). Recent fashions in the medical use of hypnotic drugs in England and Wales – the end of the barbiturate era. In Clift, A.D. (ed.), *Sleep Disturbance and Hypnotic Drug Dependence*, Amsterdam, Excerpta Medica

Parish, P.A. (1976). *Medicines: A Guide for Everybody*, Harmondsworth, Middlesex, Penguin

Parish, P.A., Stimson, G.V., Mapes, R.E.A. and Cleary, J. (1976). Prescribing in general practice. *Journal of the Royal College of General Practitioners 26*, Supplement 1

Pradal, H. (1974). *Guide des médicaments les plus courants*, Paris, Editions du Seuil

Price Commission, (1978). *Prices, Costs and Margins in the Production and Distribution of Proprietary Non-ethical Medicines*, London, HMSO

PROP (Paper of the National Prisoners' Movement) (1978). *2, 4*, London

Rabin, D.L. and Bush, P.J. (1974). The use of medicines: historical trends and international comparisons. *Int. J. Health Serv. 4*, 1, 61-87

Robinson, D. (1971). *The Process of Becoming Ill*, London, Routledge and Kegan Paul

Robinson, D. and Henry, S. (1977). *Self-help and Health*, London, Martin Robertson

Roche Products Ltd. (1968). A life of anxiety and the place of Valium Roche

Roth, J. (1978). *Health Purifiers and Their Enemies*, London, Croom Helm

Sackett, D.L. and Haynes, R.B. (1976). *Compliance with Therapeutic Regimens*, Baltimore, John Hopkins University Press

Scheff, T.J. (1963). Decision rules, types of error, and their consequences in medical diagnosis. *Behav. Sci. 8*, 97-107

Schwartz, L.R. (1969). The hierarchy of resort in curative practices: the

Admiralty Islands, Melanesia. *J. Hlth & Soc. Beh. 10*, 201-9

Stimson, G.V. (1974). Obeying doctor's orders: a view from the other side. *Soc. Sci. Med. 8*, 97-104

Stimson, G.V. and Webb, B. (1975). *Going to see the Doctor: The Consultation Process in General Practice*, London, Routledge and Kegan Paul

Stimson, G.V. (1976). Doctor-patient interaction and some problems for prescribing. In: Parish *et al.* (1976) op cit

Stimson, G.V. (1978). Treatment or control? Dilemmas for staff in drug dependency clinics. In West, D.J. (ed.), *Problems of Drug Abuse in Britain*, Cambridge, Institute of Criminology

Wadsworth, M.E.J., Butterfield, W.J.H. and Blaney, R. (1971). *Health and Sickness: The Choice of Treatment*, London, Tavistock Publications

White, K.L., Jelkovic, D., Pearson, R.J.C., Mabry, J.H., Ross, A. and Sagen, O.K. (1967). International comparisons of medical care utilisation. *New England J. Med. 277*, 516-22

Wren, R.C. (1971). *Potter's New Cyclopaedia of Botanical Drugs and Preparations*, Rushington, Sussex, Health Science Press

Zola, I.K. (1973). Pathways to the doctor: from person to patient. *Social Science and Medicine 7*, 677-89

Zola, I.K. (1976). Taking one's medicine: whose problem is it? Paper presented at Being Healthy in Boston: Is It Possible or Even Probable? Boston City Hospital, March

3 THE INTRODUCTION OF NEW DRUGS

Alex Lumbroso

Introduction

Whenever a new pharmaceutical compound is presented to a physician, he should be told its therapeutic class, pharmacological effects, mechanism of action, duration of action, administration and routes of elimination. He also needs to know about the clinical use of the drugs, its contraindications, dosage, warnings, interactions with other drugs, and the symptoms and treatment of overdosage (Herxheimer and Lionel, 1978). Information on all the pharmaceutical forms and the presentation of the drug be also available to him. He must be sure that the product is stable and of good quality.

These essential data have frequently not reached doctors and are often not all complete during the first years after the introduction of a product. Meanwhile, the more active the new drugs are, the greater the need for the required information.

This need for precise data has led to a fundamental change in the pharmaceutical industry and also in clinical research. Any product intended for therapeutic use is now subjected to 3 types of research:

(1) Its pharmacological properties are defined by standard methods used in the pharmaceutical industry laboratories. These methods must be sometimes simplified and come to be routines. The stability of the product is examined, for this will determine its shelf life. The finished product used by patients and stocked under normal conditions is investigated to detect possible degradation into toxic or inactive compounds.

(2) Toxicity and teratogenicity studies are performed in animals in order to increase the safety of clinical trials in man. Pharmacological and toxicological studies in animals are used to provide as much information as possible before pharmacokinetics and human pharmacology are investigated in healthy volunteers or patients.

(3) Only after these studies can clinical studies give information on the efficacy, the side effects and the daily dose of the drug. They can also confirm its therapeutic potential when compared to existing products on the market.

61

At the end of these long, rigorous and usually tedious studies, the company will be able to calculate the price at which the drug is to be sold and will decide whether it is to be launched into the competitive world of prescription medicines.

In reality this scheme is less simple. Consider the following limitations. Firstly, the pharmaceutical company needs to optimise its limited resources. How can this optimisation influence the development of new pharmaceutical products? Secondly, clinical research is the basic tool for the introduction of any drug and is becoming increasingly important. How should it be used and why? Thirdly, public opinion and the media are intensely interested in drugs, which in a way symbolise everyone's right to health care. How does this concern affect the introduction of new drugs? Fourthly, government regulations are relied upon to safeguard the public interest. How can such regulations influence the introduction of drugs?

These four prominent factors profoundly affect the work of those who are responsible for the development and the introduction of new pharmaceutical products. Any therapeutic progress ultimately depends on the control of these factors.

Contribution of Company Resources to the Development of New Drugs

Among the 250 or so product licences granted to new drugs each year in France, for example, 200 are for combinations of known molecules, 25 for a new formulation of a previously known active compound and 20 are for a new molecular entity. Only 5 are innovations of therapeutic interest.

Among 250 drugs, 225 are the results of development studies without previous research, and only 25 result from an attempt at innovation. This is probably because company managements find it difficult to decide, on the one hand, what resources should be allocated to research and to the development of new drugs, and, on the other hand, how they should orientate this research strategically. This difficulty has three causes:

(1) The profitability of development can be calculated but that of research cannot.
(2) The assessment of potential markets is mainly based on retrospective data.
(3) Although the product is aimed at human therapeutic needs,

the company's research is nearly always based on experimental models.

The Profitability of Development can be Calculated While that of Research Cannot

The discovery of cimetidine is the most striking example of recent years. The small team of about 25 led by J.W. Black which completed this research programme was very familiar with the academic background work on the antagonism of H_2 histamine receptors, having worked previously on related subjects. The team did not hesitate to synthesise and to select hundreds of compounds long before isolating the one which was going to be used successfully to reduce gastric acidity in the treatment of peptic ulcers. After the launch of cimetidine, Smith Kline and French reported a 45 per cent rise in turnover and a 90 per cent rise in profit.

This is not the only example. Innovations mainly in the antibiotic field have resulted in outstanding profits for companies which have sponsored them. In contrast some research centres with several hundred investigators have not for decades made any striking discovery. But since research centres must show results, they tend to develop products of fairly low innovation or of limited therapeutic interest. Such work enables them to show promising though modest results which can compare favourably with those of already exploited markets.

There are also companies which, because of their size and varied activities, cannot invest in research £2 million a year (which the National Economic Development Office estimated in 1970 was the minimum amount required). They consequently use their 'research' budget only for development.

The managing director must base his strategic choice (1) on creative people with imagination and tenacity, who are close to academic biological research or (2) on a study of potential markets, using his skill to develop products without real innovation, although the products must be likely to find a place in those markets. These two strategies are completely separate: they cannot be linked.

In the latter case, the chief executive will act as an apparently wise financial manager, while in the former case he will appear as a bold visionary, taking risks that are at best difficult to reconcile with his other responsibility as a financial manager. The wise manager will not find it easy to select what he needs.

The Assessment of Potential Markets is Mainly Based on Retrospective Data

This second difficulty explains why, for example, a score of anti-inflammatory drugs was launched in Europe during 1978. Their structures differ slightly and they were selected by the same pharmacological screening process. Their efficacy is of the same order as that of existing anti-inflammatories on the market. None of these drugs influences the course of rheumatic disease. The use of some of them in the treatment of degenerative joint disease is due more to marketing considerations than to any specific efficacy.

A study by De Haen (1978) shows that the number of drugs launched during 1976-7 was proportional to the importance of therapeutic classes shown in market research (see Table 3.1). When one looks more closely at the list of these drugs, many derivatives of propranolol, of clofibrate, and of diuretic sulphonamides can be found among the new cardiovascular products. The class of benzodiazepines can nearly always furnish 'new' CNS drugs. In any therapeutic class copies of limited innovation far outnumber genuinely new products of research.

One should not, however, underestimate the interest of the prescriber for some of these 'new' products. The diversity of antibiotics is justified because of bacterial resistance. The multiplication of corticosteroid compounds has led to products that are easier to handle. Perhaps better tolerated anti-inflammatories will be selected in the future. But most of these 'new products' are introduced for purely commercial reasons which force companies to develop these markets in order to remain competitive.

Table 3.1: Drugs launched during 1977 by therapeutic class

Cardiovascular drugs	17
CNS drugs	15
Anti-infectives	15
Anti-inflammatories	12
Cancer chemotherapy	9
Gastro-intestinal drugs	8
Hormones (topical or systemic)	6
Antihistamines	4
Anti-viral drugs	3
Bronchodilators	3
	92
Miscellaneous	22
Total	114

Other managers who are even more cautious launch under their own brand name generic products which have been originated and exploited by other companies whose patents have expired. Their task in research and development will be either to discover new less costly routes of synthesis or merely to perform the bioavailability studies which regulatory authorities now require. They may also look for 'novelty' by improving the acceptability of drugs (palatability, size of tablets etc.). It is impossible for an observer outside the company to understand even approximately how much is spent in innovative research. This impossibility is partly due to a conflict of interests which arises between the cautious manager of the company and the ambitious innovator, who tries to protect his research teams.

The American Pharmaceutical Manufacturers' Association has given (in its 18th Report, quoted in *Scrip*, 1979) precise information on the figures of research and development costs in the pharmaceutical industry: 1,266 million dollars during 1977 which account for 14 per cent of their turnover in the United States (8,900 million dollars) but still for only 8.6 per cent of the worldwide net sales achieved by the same firms (14,700 million dollars). Research and development (R and D) budgets are not broken down to show the costs of innovative research and of development, those of duplicative work required by regulatory authorities, nor can we be sure they exclude funds used to support public relations activities, including fees, etc. for advice from opinion leaders, who are useful mainly in relation to products already launched on the market.

The Pharmaceutical Company Whose Research is Aimed at Innovation is Additionally Vulnerable Because the Experimental Models are Inappropriate to the Use of Drugs in Man

The WHO guidelines for evaluation of drugs in man, issued in 1975, recommended that 'preclinical pharmacodynamic studies should be designed to demonstrate the expected therapeutic effect of a drug, and wherever practicable its mechanism. In addition such studies should be undertaken on the main systems of the body to reveal other effects of the drug desired or undesired'. Three years later in 1978, a symposium on the 'Scientific basis of official regulation of drug research and development' (De Schaepdryver et al., 1979) showed that these requirements are not always complied with. The batteries of pharmacological tests hide our ignorance about preclinical experimental models and only show a pharmacological action far removed from the desirable action in patients. Most animal experimental diseases are only distantly related to human diseases. The dose to be set for human use cannot be estimated from the therapeutic index in animals. Only human pharmacokinetic studies make it possible to select the dose.

Apart from obvious toxicity, toxicological tests present similar difficulties. Therapeutic indices recorded in animals only rarely predict the safety margin of a new compound in humans. Some idiosyncrasies found in humans will not show up. No amount of chronic toxicity studies will enable one to predict the consequences of long-term administration of a drug in the treatment of a chronic disease, the more so in patients with metabolic abnormalities.

The fact that many companies wishing to market new products work on 'me too' drugs is due to the inadequacy of animal models, which results in the elimination of many interesting chemical compounds on account of their toxicity or inefficacy. Inappropriate tests may not show the full separation of unwanted effects from the desired therapeutic properties.

The company that opts for innovative research faces an even greater obstacle than the one which has chosen merely to follow the rules of the marketplace: the clinical trials on which will depend the launch of any new product and by which its therapeutic potential will be assessed.

The Increasing Importance of Clinical Studies

However good the experimental model of a company's research team may be, and whatever the size of the research budget, these will not suffice to forecast the difficulty and the safety of a new compound in the treatment of acute or chronic human diseases. This experimental model and the clinical studies will be linked by human pharmacology studies which, because of the small number of volunteers, and because of their rigid methods, will only roughly define a theoretical dose and effective mode of administration and the likely routes of elimination of the drug. Only rigorous clinical trials can demonstrate the efficacy and acceptability of the future drug.

Irrespective of the amount of enthusiasm the research teams may have, clinical studies remain the key for product launch. But there are *three major problems*: good clinical studies are rare; rigorous long-term clinical studies in chronic diseases are extremely difficult to perform; and the company suffers if it cannot control this essential part of its research and development programme and it therefore seeks to do so. The limited availability and the importance of clinical trial facilities make them an object of intense competition among companies, and this has many consequences.

Good Clinical Trials are Rare

The method now universally recognised for evaluating the efficacy and the safety of pharmaceutical compounds is the randomised controlled clinical trial with statistically valid results. Juhl and his colleagues (1977) have examined all therapeutic trials in gastro-enterology listed in MEDLARS as published between 1964 and 1974 and have shown that this method remains an exception. Of 35,288 publications on clinical trials, randomised trials represented only 0.3 per cent of studies published in 1964 and 1.7 per cent of those published in 1974. This improvement in a decade is real, but there is still enormous scope for further improvement. Moreover, the quality of these published controlled trials could be easily criticised: most studies involved no more than 50 patients who were followed for 6 weeks. Typically, an old treatment for peptic ulcer was compared with the new compound which always proved to be superior. This critique is the only one based on a quantitative study. In France, the new chairman of the Licensing Committee for Medicines (Commission d'Autorisation de Mise sur le Marché) has stated that the introduction of the new product licence system should lead to a profound modification of clinical trials, and that even specialists in the United States have reached the same conclusions.

The guidelines for improving the methodology of clinical trials can be summarised as follows:

Phase I – Preliminary Human Studies. Efforts should be made to encourage clinical studies instead of tests on animals, which should be limited to toxicity tests and pharmacokinetics.

Protocols should spell out objectives of the study and state the specific questions the study is supposed to answer. Clinical pharmacology departments should be encouraged to expand their capacity to handle phase I studies. Institutional review committees must understand the significance of testing new therapeutic agents and be aware of the logistics of new drug development.

Phase II – First Studies in Patients. Clinicians should be encouraged to undertake clinical trials. Well-conducted trials should be recognised by academic promotion or salary increments. Reports should be made simpler and clearer.

Multicentre trials should be used when the protocol is precise and the investigators adhere to them rigidly. They should be monitored and data should be collected and reported in a uniform way. At the end of phase II, it should be decided whether the drug should be developed as a therapeutic agent.

Phase III – Clinical Trials. Trials should make it possible to clarify the relationship between any adverse reactions and the administration of a drug in single as well as in repeated doses. It is important that patients should accept the procedures of the trial and comply with them.

On the whole, these recommendations should lead to an increase of the number of 'good' clinical studies. The quality of the clinical trials can be improved in two ways. First, as Professor Legrain has stated in France, through an increasing influence of governmental agencies on the conduct of trials; second, through the development of self-discipline among members of the pharmaceutical industry, genuinely and openly supported by the leaders of the medical profession, as Johnson and Johnson (1977) conclude in their excellent book on clinical trials.

Clinical trials carried out to monitor the therapeutic value of drugs will improve technically. But how can the medical need for new drugs be assessed? Only medical need will convince the leaders of the medical profession to take part in and encourage their development. How can we cope with the fact that the number of patients available for a trial is always limited? How can we avoid psychological bias or human differences which reduce the validity of these trials?

Even when these improvements have been made and the new drug marketed, adverse reactions which cannot be investigated in clinical trials will inevitably occur, whether because of poor conditions of use, or the vulnerability of some patients, or because of prolonged use of the drug.

Rigorous Long-term Clinical Trials are Especially Difficult for Chronic Diseases

Many of the obstacles mentioned above which could be overcome are in these cases difficult to face. Should we wait for the results of a long and strict prospective study before giving anticoagulants, clofibrate or nicotinic acid, or all three drugs together, to patients with myocardial infarction? Should we rather undertake a genetic study of all patients having to take a drug chronically? It took one year's treatment for the development of retinopathy with chloroquine to be recorded and many years to analyse the finding.

The new strict methods required during the phase before marketing should certainly remain in use throughout the commercial life of a product. Long-term studies nowadays mainly aim to record metabolic variations and are often retrospective. They are not generally well controlled. Here again it is doubtful if patients are sufficiently motivated to take part in a long-term prospective study. In such studies would it be possible to autopsy patients who died before the end of the trial?

Recorded adverse reactions are not systematically examined. We have known for a long time that spontaneously recorded adverse reactions are of little value. Most efforts to systematise such reporting have failed. Progress has been made: adverse reaction registers and pharmacovigilance centres have been created, long-term studies of efficacy and adverse effects (post-marketing surveillance) have been proposed, research requirements after marketing issued — mainly for new compounds, but can a pharmaceutical company really be expected to support all these prospective studies, to both sponsor and depend on such extended epidemiological studies, while the control of its activity is based on the rhythm of its budgets and its quinquennial forecasts?

Control of Clinical Trials

The pharmaceutical company strives hard to control the clinical trials of its drugs which are an essential part of its drug development programme and which will enlarge throughout the life-span of their patents. Clinical trial facilities and the trials themselves are a strategic basic material, vital for the development of new products. They are controlled by clinicians of unequal quality, with different resources in patients. Some clinicians refuse to do trials because they wish to avoid any collaboration with pharmaceutical companies, while others live on them. They are performed not only in hospitals but also by general practitioners. The commercial future of a pharmaceutical product largely depends on the outcome of these trials throughout the life-span of the product. This basic material is so scarce, especially when it is of recognised quality, that companies fight each other for it. This struggle is based on the supply and demand system: the scarcity of good trial opportunities has led to a huge increase in the costs and duration of clinical trials.

For a middle-ranking French pharmaceutical company, the cost of human pharmacology and clinical studies accounts for 40 per cent of the total research and development budget.

The means used by the pharmaceutical firms to corner these trials and to control them are simple and classical: the large groups systematically give financial support to those specialised clinical units that will be useful for their trials; multiple similar clinical trials of little scientific interest are organised by or for the marketing department to introduce products into hospitals; prescriptions by general practitioners are in effect purchased by the organisation of multiclinic trials. This state of affairs does not help the efforts made to improve clinical trials.

Nevertheless, we should note that the movement to improve clinical trials is only 20 years old, that the leaders of the profession support it with increasing strength and that it is leading to the publication of much good work on methodology — trends which will help to widen the gap between manipulated and ill-designed clinical trials and well-controlled trials which should soon remain the only ones to be published. These forces will in due course reduce the number of new drugs to those few that bring a therapeutically useful innovation.

Pressures From Public Opinion

Two factors outside the industry play an important part in the introduction of drugs. These are, on the one hand, the consumers and public opinion and, on the other, the regulations which make the pharmaceutical industry one of the most tightly controlled industries.

It seems more constructive to analyse their participation in therapeutic progress than to criticise them and merely to clarify the industry's irrational and sometimes contradictory reactions to them.

Faced with new drugs, the public, very much aware of its right to health, has the consumer's classical reactions to any new product. But it could play a positive part by reacting in a new way to the ethics of the trials in man and also by favouring the development of drugs of apparently limited commercial interest.

(1) Companies which develop new drugs are encouraged to 'play safe' by the pressure of consumers who are increasingly using pharmaceutical products, while at the same time they are getting more and more information from the media about therapeutic accidents. Such accidents are the subject of editorials and special articles in the mass media and are immediately seized upon by consumer movements: this led to the ban on clofibrate in Germany (*Le Monde*, 1979) as well as the banning of

colouring agents elsewhere.

These movements also voice very critical reactions to the industry, which are often justified, e.g. in the case of the clioquinol and thalidomide disasters. These occur especially when it appears that consumers are being given wrong or defensive information. As Engelhart says 'let us not forget that in today's world of mass media and consumer interest, honest, unbiased and skilful reporting of medical news is as important as honest, unbiased and skilful clinical research' (Bankowski and Dunne, 1977). Public opinion is an effective brake on the development and introduction of harmful or useless drugs. But it is essentially because of this brake that industry tends to play safe, thus favouring the introduction of drugs that do little harm but also bring little innovation.

(2) The public is believed to be strongly opposed to the development of trials in man. Some opinion leaders would even want warnings to be increased, which would make it much more difficult to improve the scientific quality of clinical trials.

For example, in April 1979, at a formal session of the French Academy of Sciences, Professor Charles Dubost drew attention to the 'public's relative indifference to therapeutic trials' and suggested that randomised studies should be reserved for problems that could not be solved by clinical observation (*Quotidien du Médecin*, 1979).

This view, which goes against current thinking in clinical research, is one which will appeal to a public which is highly suspicious of trials in man. Everywhere in the world, patients' rights are defended with increasing vigour so as to reduce all unnecessary risks as much as possible. This is still truer where children are concerned. This movement is so strong that, in some cases, insurance companies refuse to cover experimenters for their clinical research activities. In these ways the public is attacking the medical profession for its casual attitude to the use of new drugs and for its alleged use of patients as guinea-pigs for the greater profit of pharmaceutical manufacturers.

How should one explain to a patient that he is participating in a randomised trial and that he may be given a placebo instead of a drug from which he expects relief? Does not a trial of that kind contradict the precepts of medical ethics?

None the less, many patients agree to participate in controlled trials as long as they are assured of the professional and human qualities of the doctors who are responsible for them. New regulations have been proposed to safeguard the patient's legitimate rights. The Declarations of Helsinki in 1964 and Tokyo in 1975 envisioned the establishment of ethics committees in all hospitals.

A public that is better informed about these matters will support therapeutic trials in man, if it feels convinced that they will improve the prevention and treatment of disease. However, this may also encourage pharmaceutical manufacturers to 'play safe' or perhaps to undertake clinical research in those countries where the public receives little information.

(3) Another widely held view is that industry develops only products likely to have a big market and has no interest in products of limited commercial potential. This is the case for drugs required to treat rare diseases, or diseases that occur predominantly in the poor countries of the third world.

The public's pressure is such that it is now common to see pharmaceutical companies develop so-called prestige products as part of their research programme. But the market for therapeutic innovations remains ill-understood. Again taking cimetidine as an example, the initial research results appeared to be of limited commercial interest, but they led to a drug which opened a huge market in gastro-enterology. In contrast research on prostaglandins has not yet resulted in any major product and it is hard to assess the future commercial prospects of the research on endorphins. This view has encouraged medical opinion leaders to take an interest in and facilitate research on drugs for rare diseases.

The developing countries constitute a major potential market and the public has drawn the attention of the pharmaceutical industry to the importance of this market for those drug-exporting countries which can supply them with cheaper products, or products that are better adapted to their needs. Here again, pressure from public opinion may encourage the development of drugs.

(4) The public plays an essential part in the evolution of regulations which, while intended to assure safety, would significantly delay the introduction of new drugs. This phenomenon is most obvious in the USA where the Food and Drug Administration has instituted the most onerous regulation in the world. In 1972, a FDA official, Mr Schmidt, stated that it would be possible to 'remedy this delay only if the public, like the Senate, admitted that a decision not to approve an important drug could be harmful to the public health as much as a decision to approve a potentially dangerous drug'.

But the public doubts the competence of doctors to handle every new active substance immediately after its introduction; it wants new drugs to be introduced in a limited way, so that their therapeutic value can be assessed more reliably than by the trials performed now.

Regulation

Medicines are among the most regulated products. All over the world it is impossible to give or sell any medicine if a governmental agency has not given an adequate authorisation (called AMM in France, CSM Approval in the UK, NDA in the USA). This can be obtained only by pharmaceutical companies which can demonstrate both the control of quality and satisfactory data showing the efficacy and reasonable safety of the product. The widespread adoption of such regulations is barely 10 years old. It is interesting to analyse how it developed and to try to forecast how it will evolve.

(1) Regulation has developed in response to pressure from public opinion in the wake of therapeutic accidents.

(2) At the same time it is originated by the public authorities wanting to organise and influence the medicines market.

(3) But regulation can also play a positive part by requiring the performance of good clinical trials and by favouring a more rigorous selection of drugs.

(4) However, regulation will progress only if a scientific consensus exists or can be achieved.

(1) In all countries, regulation began as a reaction to therapeutic accidents which aroused public opinion. Because regulations were hastily made to prevent repetition of the accidents which had led to them, they at first differed greatly from one country to another. For instance, in September and October 1937, in the USA, sulfanilamide elixir containing ethylene glycol as a solvent caused at least 73 deaths. The investigation by the US congress which followed led to the creation of the FDA.

In France since the beginning of the century, tin oxide had been used empirically to treat skin carbuncles, until in 1952, a preparation of diethyl tin diiodide of doubtful stability poisoned about 270 people and caused at least 100 deaths. Public opinion was deeply moved by this accident. As a result French regulation was changed and became more rigorous and formalistic. For example, the strict requirements for batch testing have often been considered to be a protectionist device.

All over Europe, the catastrophe caused by thalidomide in 1959-60 led to the creation of new regulatory systems. The drug was marketed everywhere except in France and in the USA, where rigid regulation had created administrative delays.

All these regulations are based on the same principle, but entail various biases which are due to: different legal customs; the scientific Committees that proposed them and which differ in composition; the uneven levels of protection of these markets against imports; and finally to pressure from the public and media. In Great Britain, for instance, a country of liberal traditions and of strong self-discipline, there was no regulation before thalidomide. In 1964, a tedious and rigorous but voluntary system of regulation was created. But though it was voluntary, all members of the ABPI (Association of the British Pharmaceutical Industries) were obliged to comply with it. In 1971 this was replaced by a statutory system of regulation. In Germany, on the other hand, the country where thalidomide was developed, no regulations were made until EEC rules were imposed in 1972.

(2) The regulation of pharmaceuticals, like all regulations, aims also to organise markets. It is often stated that France and the USA, both countries which have developed strict rules, intended by multiple and complex controls to protect their domestic pharmaceutical industry by preventing foreign companies from entering the market without the help of a domestic company. Perhaps the need to limit the cost of drugs was an additional factor in France.

It will be interesting to analyse the evolution of this system of regulation in Europe and to see how far the Committee on Proprietary Medicinal Products, which was created by a directive in 1975, will be able to implement the free circulation of drugs through the EEC countries by 1990. The rules for authorising the marketing of a drug vary considerably. The EEC Commission would prefer a common procedure while the pharmaceutical industry favours mutual recognition of national procedures. The EEC administration, wanting to organise and control the drug market, needs the agreement of the European companies. The protection of public health is probably not the only point at issue. Another important reason for these differences may be the difficulty of harmonising drug prices that are related to differences in social security systems.

As an example, Norwegian regulation is extremely restrictive. It requires the demonstration of a genuine medical need for the new drug before its introduction is authorised. According to the Norwegian public authorities, this rule is intended to reduce health costs by limiting the number of drugs available and to enable practitioners to understand existing products better while avoiding the dilution of drug information.

In Sweden very rigorous clinical trials are required before marketing is authorised and they must be replicated in the country. Such a rule could be misused for a protectionist purpose, especially when the pharmaceutical industry is publicly owned.

(3) Before the marketing of a drug is authorised, all countries require stringent clinical trials. Such trials, more than anything else, lead to a rigorous selection of new drugs. All clinicians make the same criticism of the inadequacy of clinical trials performed before the 'regulatory era'. In the past a pharmacological result was commonly equated with thera-peutic action, drug potency with drug efficacy, the number of clinical trials with their quality. Today guidelines for good clinical trials are being prepared, thanks to the influence of international organisations such as, inter alia, CIOMS (Council for International Organisations of Medical Sciences) or the Heymans Foundation (De Schaepdryver et al., 1979) or even of regulatory bodies such as the FDA or the EEC. These are randomised controlled studies, often double-blind, rather than open trials. A further step will be their organisation on an international basis. But much remains to be done. In France, for instance, regulations and the code of medical ethics both prohibit studies of clinical pharmacology and of randomised trials involving the use of a placebo. This position completely contradicts the regulations which require human pharmacokinetics and controlled trials before a product licence can be issued. Furthermore, public opinion continues to oppose clinical trials in man while demanding at the same time that authorisation to market new drugs be given only in stages, so that more is known about the drugs by the time they are made generally available. Only a scientific consensus will succeed in reconciling these contradictions.

(4) Indeed only a scientific consensus will enable the regulatory bodies to overcome certain rigid legal requirements which lead to duplication, or differences in the technical details of analytical, pharmacological, toxicological or clinical controls between the various countries.

Dr J.R. Crout, Director of the Bureau of Drugs of the Food and

Drug Administration, summarised conditions in 1978 in a paper on the acknowledgement by the American authorities of trials carried out abroad:

> I believe we must recognize the major reasons for our differences are non-scientific. They derive instead from differences in legal standards, attitudes, and the decision-making processes of government in our respective countries. I would not deny that gains can be made at the technical level from international consensus on such matters as toxicology requirements and methods of evaluation of safety and effectiveness. But only partial harmonization of approval decisions can result from such technical reconciliation.

Such a scientific consensus would enable agreement to be reached on the limits of the standards of pre-clinical and toxicological tests at the time when it would be necessary to undertake pharmacokinetic studies on man, but it would especially bring about a harmonisation of clinical trial methods and also a sharing of clinical trial resources on a wide international scale instead of only a national one.

The ideal, from the scientists' point of view, would be a unique and worldwide marketing authorisation. However, the replications still required by many countries are not all on the debit side. They will also clarify the action of new drugs, bring to light new therapeutic indications and will foster comparative studies with different products in different countries.

An example will demonstrate the importance of a scientific consensus on regulatory policies. Research on recombinant DNA which had been tightly restricted by the American regulatory authority, was permitted on a much wider scale by the National Institutes of Health at the instigation of a special committee, comprising not only scientists but also some representatives of the general public. It was also decided that the reports of this committee should be published. The advantages offered by such an approach should be understood by the regulatory authorities and by drug manufacturers as well as by the scientific community.

References

Bankowski, Z. and Dunne, J.F. (1977). Trends and prospects in drug research and development. *CIOMS* Round Table Conference *11*, December

Casadio, S. (1978). Coûts de la recherche pharmaceutique et innovation thérapeutique. *Labo-Pharma – Problèmes et Techniques 280*, 789-91

Clinical Pharmacology and Therapeutics (1975). *18*, 5, Part 2

De Schaepdryver, A.F., Gross, F.H., Lasagna, L. and Laurence, D.R. (eds.) (1979). *Scientific Basis of Official Regulation of Drug Research and Development*, Ghent, Heymans Foundation

Duchier, J. (1979). De La molécule au médicament. *La Revue du Praticien – Pédiatrie 29*, 17, 1463-8; *29*, 23, 1961-5

Euroforum (1978). La consommation pharmaceutique: une escale difficile à contrôler, *44*, 78, Annexe 1

De Haen, P. (1978). Revue biannuelle des médicaments nouveaux introduits aux Etats-Unis (1976-1977). *Labo-Pharma – Problèmes et Techniques 282*, 991-1000

Herxheimer, A. and Lionel, N.D.W. (1978). Minimum information needed by prescribers. *British Medical Journal 2*, 1129-32

Johnson, N. and Johnson, S. (1977). *Clinical Trials*, Oxford, Blackwell Scientific Publications.

Juhl, E., Christensen, E. and Tygstrup, N. (1977). The epidemiology of the gastrointestinal randomized clinical trial. *New England Journal of Medicine 296*, 20-2

Kornprobst, L. (1979). Essais des nouveaux médicaments chez l'homme. *La Nouvelle Presse Médicale 8*, 1531-4

Lahon, H., Rondel, R.K. and Kratochivil, C. (eds.) (1979). *Pharmaceutical Medicine: the Future*, Brussels, Acta Therapeutica

Le Monde (1979). Clofibrate, maladies métaboliques et préventions cardio-vasculaires. *17*

Quotidien du Médecin (1979). Les essais thérapeutiques n'intéressent pas assez le public. *1903*, 8, Avril

Reekie, D. (1978). Recherche et Industrie. S'adapter à l'évolution du monde. *Prospective et Santè 7*, 93-107

Scrip (1979). No. 352, 24 January, 12

4 THE PROMOTION OF PRESCRIPTION DRUGS AND OTHER PUZZLES[1]

Milton Silverman and Mia Lydecker

In 1974, a study was undertaken on the manner in which multinational pharmaceutical companies were promoting identical products to physicians in the United States and to those in ten Latin American countries – Mexico, Guatemala, El Salvador, Honduras, Nicaragua, Costa Rica, Panama, Colombia, Ecuador, and Brazil. To some of us, the differences were unbelievable. To some, they were sickening.[2]

In the United States, where promotion is under the rigid control of the Food and Drug Administration, the indications or claims of efficacy were usually few in number and limited to those that could be supported by convincing scientific evidence. Warnings, contraindications, and potential adverse reactions were disclosed in detail. Since the passage of the so-called Kefauver-Harris Amendments in 1962, this has been required by law. In Latin America, however, the situation is startlingly different. In most instances, claims of efficacy were grossly exaggerated, and warnings were minimised, glossed over, or totally omitted.

In the case of Parke-Davis' chloramphenicol (Chloromycetin), for example, physicians in the United States had long been warned that this potent and unquestionably effective antibiotic should be used only in such life-threatening infections as typhoid fever, Rocky Mountain spotted fever, Haemophilus influenzae meningitis and a few other conditions in which no safer drug was available. Large type was used in such publications as *Physicians' Desk Reference (PDR)* to warn physicians against prescribing the drug for trivial infections. But in Latin America, the product was openly recommended for such scarcely life-threatening conditions as tonsillitis, pharyngitis, bronchitis, urinary tract infections, ulcerative colitis, pneumonia, staphylococcus infections, streptococcus infections, yaws and gonorrhoea. A competitive brand, marketed by McKesson, was recommended for whooping cough.

Physicians in the United States were warned that the use of chloramphenicol may result in serious or fatal aplastic anaemia and other blood dyscrasias. Similar warnings were given to physicians for the Parke-Davis product in Mexico, but not to those in Central America. McKesson's Chloramfenicol MK was accompanied by warnings in

Central America but not in Colombia and Ecuador. No potential adverse reactions were given for another competitive brand, Winthrop's Wintetil.

Similar discrepancies were found with most of some two dozen different drugs marketed in the form of 40 different products by 23 multinational companies based in the United States, Switzerland, France and West Germany.

When these discrepancies were called to the attention of the companies, most were unable to explain them. More important, spokesmen for most firms expressed no interest in correcting the situation.

Our findings were published in May 1976. By September of the same year, roughly one-half of the multinational firms involved had already changed their labelling and promotion policies in Latin America, and were telling essentially the same story to all physicians. In December, the council of the International Federation of Pharmaceutical Manufacturers Associations adopted by unanimous vote a US- introduced resolution calling for essentially standardised drug labelling worldwide with full disclosure of hazards.

An account of some of the events leading up to these developments may indicate how an informed and aroused public, in developed and underdeveloped nations alike, along with socially responsible physicians and scientists within the drug companies themselves, can take effective action to improve the quality of health care in general and drug promotion in particular.

The Chloramphenicol Record

For a number of reasons, the record of chloramphenicol has long held a particular fascination for students of drug marketing and promotion. Introduced by Parke-Davis as Chloromycetin in 1949, it was quickly recognised as an important and remarkably effective antibiotic. By 1952, however, it had also become evident that it could cause fatal aplastic anaemia and other blood disorders. In the United States, some physicians felt the drug should be taken off the market, but the Food and Drug Administration (FDA) — after careful consultation with the National Research Council and a nationwide panel of experts — decided it should remain available, but only for cautious use in potentially fatal conditions, in which no other antibiotic was effective.

From 1952 to 1967, the FDA, the *Journal of the American Medical*

Association, and other medical publications continued to issue warnings against the indiscriminate use of chloramphenicol, and Parke-Davis continued to intensify its promotion, extolling the product and minimising its hazards. Its detail men were instructed not to mention toxicity 'unless the physician brings up the subject'. At hearings of a US Senate subcommittee, Senator Gaylord Nelson – long a forceful critic of drug industry promotional activities – took Parke-Davis officials to task for failing to disclose the hazards of chloramphenicol in foreign countries.

'We are breaking no laws', a company spokesman retorted. 'Disclosure of hazards is not required in those other countries.' Such a defence seemed airtight. There was nothing that could be done by the Congress or FDA to control the foreign promotion of US-based firms.

But not all Americans stood by. In Southern California, ten-year-old James Watkins died from aplastic anaemia after Chloromycetin had been given to him for a urinary tract infection by two physicians – one of them his own father, Dr Albe Watkins.

Afterwards, Dr Watkins presented the following testimony before a Senate hearing:

This drug was given to me by a representative of Parke-Davis . . . This man told me there were no reactions, this was a perfectly safe antibiotic. So I took the drug home and placed it in my medicine cabinet.

A few days later, my son suffered a urinary tract infection, and I went to the cabinet and looked at the drugs I had. I picked up a bottle of sulfa, and I said, I don't want to give him this, because this might depress his bloodmaking system. Imagine that! And I looked at Aureomycin and Terramycin, and I said, sometimes this upsets the stomach, and I don't want him to get sick with the drug. And then I spotted the Chloromycetin. And I gave him the Chloromycetin, which caused his death several months later. A druggist, about two blocks from my office, asked me, 'How did you happen to give him Chloromycetin?' And I said, 'This is the one drug that I thought was harmless.'

The pharmacist told me, 'I told the representative three days before that, that the drug was harmful, that a lady had died in Pasadena' . . . So the representative of Parke-Davis knew at the time he gave me the drug, he deliberately lied to me that the drug was harmless.

This representative of Parke-Davis was given a three months' leave of absence. He later sold his home and moved out of the area. I understand his health was not too good after that.

Almost the same tragedy struck 5-year-old Mary Patricia Corcoran, the daughter of an Indiana physician, and 20-year-old Brenda Lynne Elfstrom, daughter of the publisher of a small California newspaper. Both victims had been given the drug for a minor infection.

The parents of these three victims took it upon themselves to embark on a crusade. They travelled back and forth across the country – at their own expense – and talked personally to physicians, pharmacists, and newspaper editors wherever they could. They testified before legislative committees. They denounced Parke-Davis' 'we're breaking no laws' defence as immoral, unethical, and socially irresponsible.

Perhaps the most active crusaders were Professor and Mrs Alvin Zander of Michigan, whose daughter had died from aplastic anaemia after being treated in Spain for a sore throat. She had been given what was probably, though not proved to be, Parke-Davis' Chloromycetin. The Zanders travelled repeatedly to Europe, collecting evidence of the overzealous promotion of the drug, and demanding action from the US government, from foreign ministries of health, and from Parke-Davis itself. Mrs Zander appeared at stockholder meetings of the company and pleaded for full disclosure of hazards, but the stock-holders were apparently appeased by company statements that 'we're breaking no laws.'

Oddly, the stand of the company officers was not unanimous. While those concerned with marketing and sales insisted on maintaining the policy of covering up on hazards, those involved with research and medical affairs – some of them, at least – tried year after year to change that policy, but without notable effects.

The Latin American Research

Our own study began in 1974, after we had published a report on how prescription drugs in the United States are discovered, produced, promoted, priced, prescribed by physicians and used by patients – and how these potent products are too frequently mispromoted, mis-prescribed and misused. We had not yet examined the situation in other countries. One morning at a seminar at the University of California School of Medicine, where our work was being discussed, a young physician from San Diego offered what was destined for us to be a fateful suggestion: 'If you think the companies have done such a miserable job of promotion in the United States', he said, 'you should see what they're still doing in Mexico'. 'What are they doing in Mexico?' He said, 'You wouldn't believe it. Go look for yourself.' We[3] decided to look and not only in Mexico.

The study was based on a comparison of the promotional or labelling material on 40 different products marketed by the same multinational company or its foreign affiliates in Mexico, Central America, Colombia, Ecuador, and Brazil. The volume used for the United States was the latest available edition of *Physicians' Desk Reference*. It was chosen as the basis for the comparative study, not because its statements are necessarily valid or acceptable to all physicians, pharmacists, and drug companies, but because the statements in *PDR* are based on material that has been formally approved by a federal agency, they are at least tolerable to most drug manufacturers, and the book is widely distributed to all practising physicians, and frequently consulted by them. Under existing laws, the *PDR* statements — considered to be both labelling and promotion, or a form of paid advertising — must include not only claims of efficacy but also warnings, contraindications, and potential adverse reactions. The comparable 1973 volumes for the Latin American countries were these:

For Mexico: *Diccionario de Especialidades Farmacéuticas Edición Mexicana*;
For the Central American countries and also the Dominican Republic: *Diccionario de Especialidades Farmacéuticas, Edición CAD*;
For Ecuador and Colombia: *Diccionario de Especialidades Farmacéuticas, Edicion E Co.*;
For Brazil: *Index Terapêutico Moderno*.

The material in these Latin American reference works was not approved by any governmental agency. The claims made for each product were those that the manufacturer wanted to make, and the hazards disclosed — if any — were those that the manufacturer wanted to disclose.

In addition to chloramphenicol, the survey covered other antibiotics, oral contraceptive products, non-steroid antiarthritics, steroid hormones, antipsychotic tranquillisers, antidepressants, and anticonvulsants.

Some of the findings are indicated here.

Antibiotics. In the United States, the description of Lederle's tetra-
cycline (Achromycin or Acromicina) included extensive warnings of the
possibility of interference with bone and tooth development in
children, liver damage, and overgrowth of non-susceptible organisms.
In the comparable reference volumes in Mexico, Central America and
Brazil, such matters were mentioned only briefly or not at all.

Serious adverse reactions, particularity ototoxicity, caused by
Schering's gentamicin (Garamycin or Garamicina) were described
in detail in the United States but minimised or dismissed as 'rare'
in Latin America.

Serious or potentially fatal side effects of Squibb's fungizone
(Fungizon or Amfostat) were spelled out in detail in the United States
but minimised or not mentioned in the other countries.

Oral Contraceptives. For all such products marketed in the United
States, the only accepted use was for the prevention of pregnancy
(except for a high-dosage form approved for the control of
endometriosis and hypermenorrhoea). Physicians were warned of the
risk of serious and potentially fatal thromboembolic changes.

In Latin America, these products were recommended not only for
contraception but also for the control of pre-menstrual tension,
dysmenorrhoea, the problems of the menopause and a host of other
conditions. No warnings of adverse reactions were given for Searle's
Ovulen or Wyeth's Ovral or Anfertil in Ecuador, Colombia, or Brazil,
or Parke-Davis' Norlestrin or Prolestrin in Central America. The
descriptions of Syntex's Norinyl in the United States and Mexico,
however, were essentially the same.

Non-steroid Antiarthritics. Ciba-Geigy's phenylbutazone (Butazolidina)
and an 'alka' product combining the drug with an antacid were
described to physicians in the United States as products that are not
to be considered simple analgesics or administered casually. They have
limited indications, usually severe forms of certain specified arthritic
conditions. They may cause stomach or duodenal ulcer, sometimes
with perforation, and a serious or fatal blood dyscrasia. They are
contraindicated in children and in senile patients. Especially in the
elderly, treatment should be limited to brief periods.

In striking contrast, Latin American physicians were advised that
these products are useful not only in serious arthritic conditions but
also in a wide variety of conditions marked by fever, pain, and
inflammation. The 'alka' form was described as 'especially indicated

for patients with sensitive stomachs and prolonged treatments, as well as in infancy, adolescence and advanced age'. In some countries, no contraindications, warnings, or adverse reactions were mentioned.

Similar discrepancies were observed in the case of McKesson's Fenilbutazona MK.

Steroid Hormones. Four widely used corticosteroid hormones were included in the study: Schering's prednisone (Meticorten) and betamethasone (Celestone), Lederle's triamcinolone (Aristocort or Ledercort), and Upjohn's methylprednisolone (Medrol). All of these, especially if used for excessive periods, may cause unpleasant or deadly side effects, including a flare-up of latent tuberculosis, osteoporosis, vertebral compression fractures, peptic ulcer with perforation and haemorrhage, psychic changes, and many others.

Few of these hazards, however, were disclosed for Meticorten in Latin America and none for Celestone in Central America, Ecuador, Colombia, or Brazil. For both Aristocort and Medrol, the major hazards were glossed over or given in non-specific terms.

It is worthy of note that the differences were not between the United States on the one hand and Latin America on the other. Instead there were striking differences within Latin America, with the same product described by the same manufacturer in one way in Mexico, in another in Central America, and perhaps in still another in Ecuador and Colombia. In some instances, competing brands of the same drug were described differently in the same country. If there were corporate or national patterns or policies to explain these variations, they were not readily discernible.

Further, Latin America has not been singled out for such treatment by multinational companies. At least in the case of chloramphenicol, comparable differences have been apparent in such nations as France, Italy, Spain, Australia, and New Zealand (Dunne *et al.*, 1973).

In Latin America, the problem has been further complicated by the ready availability of 'prescription drugs' without a prescription. Although the practice may be illegal, it is customary for patients to obtain most drugs – with the exception of narcotics and some psychoactive agents – without a prescription of any kind. The patient may go directly to a pharmacist, or an untrained pharmacist's assistant and ask for a drug by name. Or the patient may describe the symptoms and the pharmacist will then diagnose, prescribe and dispense, often basing his decision on the promotional material distributed by the manufacturer.

The clinical results of this irrational use of drugs, whether by a pharmacist or a physician using inadequate labelling information, are difficult to measure. Among Latin American medical authorities — especially haematologists, pathologists and other experts — the damage caused by drugs is believed to be shockingly high. However, in countries where a large proportion of the population never reaches medical care, let alone a hospital with a haematology laboratory, many practitioners may be unaware of such damage.

Included in the tragic toll are the serious or fatal reactions caused by chloramphenicol and other antibiotics, the agranulocytosis and other blood dyscrasias related to excessive use of phenylbutazone and similar antiarthritics, the temporary or permanent brain damage resulting from overuse of antipsychotic tranquillisers, the life-threatening hypertensive crises that can occur with the irrational combination of two antidepressants, and the explosive flare-ups of tuberculosis, candidiasis and other infections after prolonged use of steroids. In addition, where antibiotics are excessively promoted and excessively used, the result may be the appearance of drug-resistant strains of organisms and the spread of epidemics from one nation to another, afflicting both natives and visiting tourists. The havoc created by these resistant strains has been described in recent years in Mexico, Guatemala, Egypt and the United States.

The Industry's Responses

The discrepancies in Latin American drug promotion, and especially the failure to make full disclosure of hazards, could scarcely be denied. Instead, company spokesmen have used a variety of arguments to defend their practices.

'Things are Different in Latin America.' The meaning of this argument is not clear. Perhaps it derives from a belief that life is considered to be cheap in the Third World countries.

'It's Accepted Business Practice.' Thus, as a Latin American drug promotion expert explained it, if your competitor claims five indications for his product, you should claim at least six. And if he discloses three adverse reactions, you are senseless if you disclose more than two.

'Physicians are Already Aware of the Hazards.' This argument may be counted on to infuriate drug experts and medical educators, who have witnessed all too many examples of irrational and dangerous prescribing.

'It is the Detail Man who Explains the Hazards to Physicians.' But, in Latin America as in the United States, it is commonly said that 'you don't expect a salesman to knock his own product'.

The role and importance of the detail man, or *visitador*, in Latin America remains a curious aspect of drug promotion. In the United States, in 1974 and 1975, it was estimated that there were about 24,000 detail men who regularly called on some 250,000 practising physicians, or a ratio of one detail man to about ten doctors. In contrast, there were roughly 640 detail men for 2,000 physicians in Guatemala, 9,000 detail men for 32,000 physicians in Mexico and 14,100 detail men for 45,000 practising physicians in Brazil — a ratio in those countries of approximately one to 3. Many and perhaps most detail men have completed only a secondary education. Further, it is estimated that in Latin America, the average detail man makes a bigger income, part salary and part commission, than does the average physician.

'The Discrepancies in Drug Promotion are Merely Honest Differences in Opinion.' A company spokesman may say, 'We have in our files a wealth of convincing evidence to show that our product is safe and effective for the conditions we claim. Unfortunately, the evidence is not convincing to FDA. What we have here, therefore, is a dispute between honest scientists.'

Such an argument might be more palatable if the company did not say one thing in the United States, where it is under the constant scrutiny of FDA, and another thing throughout Latin America, where perhaps the rules are less formidable. 'But', says a Colombian health official, 'when we find the company tells one story in Bogota, another in Brasilia, another in Guatemala City, and still another in Mexico City, that is difficult to comprehend.'

'Whatever Else you may Think, we are not Breaking any Laws.' The companies insist their foreign operations are directed by nationals of the country who are familiar with the laws and regulations and who abide by them. This defence seemed to be airtight in earlier US Senate hearings and meetings of company stockholders. Copies of

Latin American drug laws were not readily available in this country.

In 1975, it became possible to make on-site studies in Mexico, Guatemala, Costa Rica, Ecuador and Colombia, obtain copies of the laws, and discuss them with local government officials and attorneys. For the other countries, invaluable help was offered by Edgar Elfstrom, the Californian newspaper publisher whose daughter had been one of the first victims who died from chloramphenicol-induced aplastic anaemia. Through his intervention and that of Rodney Beaton, president of United Press International in New York, we were able to draw on the Latin American network of UPI correspondents and get quick, accurate information that otherwise would have been unavailable to us. The situation seemed to be as follows:

(1) In some countries, the company arguments were apparently true. No laws or regulations were being violated, because no rules covering drug promotion were in existence.

(2) In others, the situation was confusing. It was evident that governmental health agencies had been given legal authority to require full disclosure of hazards to all physicians, but, for whatever the reason, had elected not to apply that authority.

(3) But in still others, notably Honduras, Panama, El Salvador, and Colombia, company assertions of innocence were apparently not true. The medical promotion was in violation of laws requiring disclosure of hazards. In at least some instances the companies had been lying.

Our findings were published on 26 May 1976 as *The Drugging of the Americas*. At the same time, on the invitation of Senator Gaylord Nelson, we testified for two days on our findings before the Senate Subcommittee on Monopoly. Also testifying were Dr Philip R. Lee of the University of California, San Francisco and a former Assistant Secretary for Health; Dr Myron Wegman, former Dean of the School of Public Health of the University of Michigan, with many years experience in international health matters; George Squibb; and Robert Ledogar, formerly at the Consumers Union and then at the United Nations.

At the end of the first morning of testimony, we asked ourselves two questions:

(1) How many years would it take — four? five? six? — for our efforts to have some visible impact?

(2) What would be the immediate response of the Pharmaceutical Manufacturers Association? Among its members were some of the multinational companies whose activities we had examined.

The second question was answered immediately. In a statement issued to the press that afternoon, the PMA President, C. Joseph Stetler, said, 'We recognise the importance of the questions raised by the various witnesses appearing before the subcommittee. It is particularly important that they pointed out the complexity of the matter, and the need for transnational attention'. Discussions, he said, would be initiated with international drug associations. Within a few hours, there were further visible impacts. Newspaper accounts appeared in such influential newspapers as the *Washington Post*, the *New York Times*, the *New York Daily News*, and the *Los Angeles Times* – and, more importantly, in such publications as *Excelsior* in Mexico City, *El Tiempo* in Bogota, *Jornal de Brasil* in Rio de Janeiro, *Estado* in Sao Paulo, *Prensa* in San Salvador, and *Excelsior* and *Nacion* in San Jose, Costa Rica.

Regrettably but predictably, most of the press ire was turned against US-based global corporations. In fact, however, the villains, if villains they were, also included firms based in Switzerland, France, and West Germany. Furthermore, the promotional activities of British, Dutch, Italian, Scandinavian and even Latin American firms were not visibly superior. Many of these companies, too, exaggerated claims and concealed dangers.

Three weeks after the Senate hearings and the publication of our report, the United States delegation appeared at a meeting of the council of the International Federation of Pharmaceutical Manufacturers Associations, the group representing practically all major drug manufacturers in the world, and called for consistent disclosure of appropriate information in drug labelling, in accord with the laws and regulations of individual nations. The council was receptive. It invited the US delegation to present a formal resolution for consideration at the next meeting. In December of 1976, in Bermuda, the US delegation introduced a resolution, calling for prescription drug labelling to be consistent with 'the body of scientific and medical evidence pertaining to that product'. Moreover, 'particular care should be taken that essential information as to medical products' safety, contraindications and side effects is appropriately communicated'. The resolution was approved by unanimous vote.

The IFPMA action was merely a recommendation, and was not

binding on its members. Even before the resolution was approved, nevertheless, there were signs that individual companies were acting on their own. By September 1976, the new Central American edition of the drug reference volume went to press. These were the highlights:

> Of 26 products under investigation in our study, two had already made honest disclosure in the 1973 edition and continued to do so in 1976.
> Eleven products were described with exaggerated claims and minimised hazards in 1973, and were similarly described in 1976.
> Four companies elected to solve the problem by the expedient of not publishing anything about them in the 1976 edition.
> But for nine products, the statements had been changed, with claims limited and hazards disclosed. The manufacturers were saying to Latin American physicians essentially the same thing they were saying to physicians in the United States.

In addition, other US-based global drug companies have informed us informally that by early 1977, they were well along in rewriting their promotional and labelling material, and would soon be saying the same thing worldwide. For example, Harris Hollin, the president of one pharmaceutical firm, Lemmon Pharmacal, notified the IFPMA that it was accepting the Federation's recommendation and had decided to use US labelling and package inserts for the products it exports to more than 20 countries:

> This has caused some concern among our distributors and representatives because of the lack of this practice among their competitors in their countries . . . Notwithstanding the present competitive disadvantage, we plan to persist in this practice and are hopeful that eventually the larger companies with whom we compete will also follow this enlightened practice.

Much of the credit for these developments belongs to the members of the public who fought for years to get honest drug promotion: the representatives of consumer groups; the press, especially the Latin American press which not merely reported the facts to readers but editorially called for change; the scientists and physicians within the drug companies who worked devotedly to improve the policies of their own firms; Senator Nelson and his staff, who have long kept a merciless spotlight on drug promotion; and the top leadership of the

Pharmaceutical Manufacturers Association in Washington, DC, who at a crucial moment, stood up for social responsibility.

Other Puzzles

There are other aspects of international drug marketing that call for investigation and action. For example, in some areas, particularly in the Third World, global companies are continuing to market products that were ousted from the United States, the United Kingdom and other countries as unsafe or ineffective, or that were never accepted. In some countries, it remains to be determined whether limited health funds could be more prudently invested in improved sanitation, protection of water supplies, better nutrition, and insect control rather than in the purchase of costly drug products.

It remains to be determined whether new and tighter laws and regulations on drug promotion and quality control can be effectively implemented, or if they will be circumvented by bribery, corruption and fraud. Will physicians be guided by new and more accurate drug labelling, or will they be influenced only by the persuasive sales presentations of detail men?

The amazing differences in drug prices, sometimes high in rich countries and low in poor countries, but sometimes low in rich countries and high in poor countries, call for justification. Should underdeveloped countries, if only to conserve their financial resources, move in the direction of nationalising their drug industries? How would such nationalisation affect the development of new and improved drugs for the future?

For countries in which the largest purchaser of drugs is a national social security system, does the failure to buy high-quality, low-cost generic-name products on competitive bid instead of high-cost brand-name products represent a needless waste of funds?

It is our belief that the unforgivable practice of dumping out-dated products, those whose shelf-life has expired, on an under-developed country is no longer so common. There is, nevertheless, a feeling among drug experts in Latin America and perhaps other parts of the world that their countries do not have adequate testing facilities to assure high product quality. Does this call for the creation of an international drug testing institution, or for a certification programme with incentives and heavy penalties for individual companies?

In many parts of the world, government officials feel they
do not have adequate authority, or even adequate information, to
ban the marketing of products that are widely regarded to be
unsafe.

In some countries, needed drugs are unavailable simply because
money is unavailable. But sometimes, as we have seen in parts of
India, North Africa and remote sections of Latin America, drugs
are not available because trucks are unavailable, or roads become
impassable, or refrigeration is inadequate and they deteriorate whilst
stored in a warehouse.

Each country, including the advanced nations, must determine
for itself whether it is really essential for acceptable health care to
provide, purchase, or permit the marketing of all drugs simply
because they are offered for sale. In the United States, for instance,
clinical pharmacologists, drug economists, and third-party
administrators are already questioning the need to make available
— often at high price — 200 antibiotic or antibacterial products,
100 antihypertensive agents, 40 or 50 sedative or hypnotic products
and scores of major and minor tranquillisers. Is it desirable and
possible, perhaps by means of a national formulary, to restrict the
numbers of drug products in use, probably to the disadvantage of
a few patients but to the clinical and economic advantage of many?
Is such an approach culturally acceptable?

A related problem concerns the need for a cost-benefit analysis
of using some high-risk drugs. Thus, it may be decided that a particular
population group will benefit in the long run from widespread use of
chloramphenicol. This seems to be the situation in the People's
Republic of China, where the drug has, at least until recently, been
widely used, with full knowledge of its dangers. Presumably this use
came from a high-level decision that saving many thousands of lives
from enteric infections would justify the loss of a few lives from
aplastic anaemia.

In many countries, pharmacists will undoubtedly continue to
diagnose and prescribe, legally or not, serving as 'physicians to the
poor' and sometimes to the not-so-poor. Rarely have they had
adequate clinical training, especially in the field of diagnosis. Should
they receive additional and more intensive training in schools of
pharmacy so they can recognise the most common forms of illness
that do not require the attention of a physician, as well as those that
clearly demand physician care? Should they be given training in the
long-term care of chronic disease, as is already being provided in some

developed nations? Should the drug industry take a more active role in furnishing up-to-date information to pharmacists?

Here, as in many other areas concerning drugs, decisions must come from the populations concerned. Neither the United States nor any other country has a mandate to impose its own drug policies on a foreign nation. There certainly must be no attempt to export the Food and Drug Administration to our neighbours. If anything is to be exported, it should be drug information, which must be disseminated fully through the medical and scientific community.

The standardisation of drug labelling discussed in this chapter marks one step in what would seem to be the proper direction.

Notes

1. The research on which this chapter is based was supported in part by grants from the Janss Foundation, Los Angeles, and the Ford Foundation, New York.
2. Material in this chapter was presented, in part, to the International Conference Against Drug-Induced Sufferings, Kyoto, Japan, April 1979.
3. The editorial 'we' used throughout this chapter refers not only to the authors. It also includes Philip R. Lee, MD, of the University of California, San Francisco; Aida LeRoy, Pharm. D, and a host of physicians, pharmacists, pharmacologists, drug economists, attorneys, and government officials in the United States and Latin America, all of whom gave fully of their time, counsel and support.

References

Full bibliographical references are given in Silverman, M. (1975). *The Drugging of the Americas*, Berkeley, California, University of California Press.

Readers may wish to consult such other sources as the following:

Barnet, R.J. and Müller, R.E. (1974). *Global Reach: The Power of the Multinational Corporations*, New York, Simon and Schuster
Dunne, M., Herxheimer, A., Newman, M. and Ridley, H. (1973). Indications and warnings about chloramphenicol. *Lancet 2*, 731, October 6
Jacoby, E.M. and Hefner, D.L. (1971). Domestic and foreign prescription drug prices. *Social Security Bulletin 34*, 15, May
Ledogar, R.J. (1976). *Hungry for Profits*, New York, IDOC, North America
Silverman, M. (1977). The epidemiology of drug promotion. *International Journal of Health Services 7*, 157
Silverman, M. and Lee, P.R. (1974). *Pills, Profits and Politics*, Berkeley, California, University of California Press

5 INFORMATION AND EDUCATION ABOUT DRUGS

Georges Peters

Different groups of people manipulate drugs before they actually enter into the bodies of those whom we shall call consumers. These groups are described in other chapters of this book. Evidently, everybody who is concerned with the manufacturing, licensing, distribution, prescribing, administration and, finally, use of the drugs should have some information about them. This statement is a truism since it applies to all goods which are manufactured, distributed and, finally, consumed. Drugs, however, are among the goods on which more information is required, in order to avoid damage to the last link in the chain, the consumer.

It is also evident that *preventing damage* and, if possible, ensuring *benefit* to the consumer is the primary interest of the consumer himself, prescribing physicians, health personnel concerned with the administration of drugs and the licensing authorities, but not necessarily of other links in the chain, whose primary interests may be economic; although continued economic benefit from drugs should, but does not necessarily, depend on the absence of damage to, and the obtaining of some benefit by, the consumer.

The term 'drugs' is used here in the sense of medicaments, i.e. drugs used in therapeutic and preventive medicine. Drugs used mainly for diagnostic purposes will not be considered. Drugs used for other purposes and possessing defined, usually detrimental, effects on the human organism are called 'toxic agents' and will not be considered. Finally, we shall not consider the needs for information of manufacturers and commercial distributors.

The decision that a given drug should be used in order to prevent, cure or manage an illness or disease, or to eliminate a troublesome symptom, is taken by many people who hold a 'power of decision' which differs greatly according to their social position and function. Evidently, the information about drugs offered to a given individual should be, but rarely is, proportionate to his power of decision in the use of drugs. The power of decision may or may not be proportionate to the basic training of the decision-makers in the science of drugs.

Thus, legislators and government officials who hold a very large power of decision do not tend to be well trained in the field of drugs, but, fortunately or unfortunately, also tend to rely on the judgement of experts. The power of decision of physicians depends on their social function. As experts or when they are in charge of clinical trials, or as teachers in medical schools or in the training of medical auxiliaries, physicians have a greater power of decision than as ordinary prescribers and should possess more information. Similarly, nurses or medical auxiliaries may act as distributors of prescribed medicines, or as prescribers. They may, however, also be responsible for ordering the drugs for a dispensary or for a health centre; their larger power of decision in this role, which unfortunately often is not matched by more extensive information on drugs, may or may not be limited by restrictive lists of drugs established by authorities with a greater power of decision.

The consumer's power of decision is limited to the choice to take or not to take the drug prescribed and provided, or to purchase or not to purchase a drug prescribed or recommended by other people. These decisions tend to be taken on the basis of thoughts or feelings quite unrelated to any information on drugs which a (potential) consumer may possess.

Needs for and Distribution of Information on Drugs

Physicians as Prescribers

The needs of the medical profession for drug information have also been discussed elsewhere in this book (see Chapter 4). No physician should ever prescribe or administer a drug on which he is not thoroughly informed. Once he has by a, hopefully rational, process decided to use a drug, he should seek to obtain, recall or confirm his information on the drug. Ideally, he should remember it by its international non-proprietary name, or at least by a national non-proprietary name. His minimum information should comprise knowledge of the following:

(1) the pharmacological effects and, if relevant, the mechanisms of action of the drug;
(2) its absorption, distribution, metabolism and excretion;
(3) the usefulness of the drug against the condition to be treated or the symptom to be eliminated;
(4) the established *merit* of the drug as compared to that of other drugs used for the same purpose and to that of other therapeutic

procedures;
(5) the contraindications of the drug;
(6) possible dangers of the drug under particular physiological
or pathological conditions;
(7) adverse effects on organ systems; and
(8) the known clinically relevant drug interactions.

Furthermore, the prescriber must be informed on:

(9) the range of useful and tolerated doses for his patient, the
usual dosing interval, the average duration of treatment; and
(10) on changes of the usual dose required by particular conditions,
such as impairment of renal or biliary excretion or of metabolism,
etc.;
(11) in the interest of his patient and of the community, physicians
should also be informed on the cost of the use of drugs.

Since all drugs may, occasionally, be taken in doses other than those
prescribed, either inadvertently or with suicidal intent, prescribers
should be familiar with:

(12) the symptoms of poisoning by overdoses and the treatment of
such poisoning.

Finally, before prescribing a drug, a physician must be informed on
the dosage forms available, on the strength of dosage forms, on the
package sizes and on the legal requirements for prescribing a drug.
He, furthermore, should be informed on the 'excipients' contained
in the particular product which he prescribes, not only because of
possible allergic effects of these ingredients, but also because of the
possibility of toxic effects of excipients and of interactions of
excipients with the drug prescribed or with other drugs currently
taken by the patient; this, however, is an ideal requirement which is
rarely, if ever, fulfilled.

In contrast, however, it is less important for a prescribing physician
to know the name and address of the manufacturer or importer of a
drug on which he is usually informed. Some knowledge of storage
conditions and expiry dates is useful but is not a primary requirement
in countries where the physician can rely on some help from dispensing
pharmacists.

The minimum information required by a physician who wishes

to prescribe a drug has been summarised in papers concerned with the development of drug information sheets containing the minimum information for physicians on a given drug (see Hollister, 1974; Herxheimer, 1974; Herxheimer and Lionel, 1978; WHO, 1977). Minimum information on a drug which a physician should possess must be completed by minimum information on the disease or symptom to be treated and on the patient for whom the drug is prescribed.

The physician must be informed on the maximal possible benefits for the consumer, which he must compare with the maximal possible discomfort or damage which could be induced by adverse reactions or interactions with other drugs, or other chemicals. This information is usually not produced on extensive (drug labels or scientific drug information sheets) or abbreviated (stuffers or package inserts) drug information sheets and must be sought or confirmed in textbooks or articles on therapeutics. Furthermore, in order to prescribe a drug rationally, the physician must be fully informed on his patient's previous pathological and allergic history.

Analogous requirements apply to drugs given for preventive purposes. The frequent occurrence of drug-induced disease in highly developed countries (Gardner and Watson, 1970; Davies, 1977) suggests that physicians often prescribe drugs without possessing the minimum information outlined above.

There are a number of reasons why physicians may, and apparently sometimes do, prescribe drugs on which they are inadequately informed:

(1) Adverse effects of a drug or adverse interactions with other drugs given to a patient may not have been observed previously. This danger exists, of course, to a particularly large extent for new drugs and can be obviated only by measures which discourage the introduction of new drugs unless they meet stringent requirements in respect to the risk/benefit ratio. A 'rapid renewal of the therapeutic armamentarium' may present considerable economic advantage to producers and distributors but carries risks to the health of individuals (and the economics of communities) which so far have not been adequately evaluated. In our opinion, minimum information for prescribing physicians on drugs used for less than 3 to 5 years should include a full description of potential adverse effects and interactions that can be predicted from the chemical nature of the new compound and its initial study in laboratory animals.

The adverse interactions of both old and new drugs comprise those with environmental chemicals which fail to be described or even suspected, because the nature of the environmental chemicals to which a particular human being is exposed is usually unknown to the physician as well as to the consumer.

(2) Information on detrimental effects or interactions or the absence of a therapeutic benefit of a drug may be available in principle but may not have been published. This is undoubtedly a frequent occurrence. Adverse drug reactions, unrelated to the basic pharmacological effects of a drug are usually not discovered in the major trials which precede marketing of a drug. Physicians who first observe adverse reactions, of course, usually cannot be sure if damage observed in a patient can really be attributed to a drug: they, therefore, usually hesitate to publish their ambiguous observations. When physicians are prepared to write to anyone about a suspected adverse drug reaction, they will usually write to the manufacturer, who may or may not feel compelled to inform licensing authorities or other doctors. Adverse reaction alarm systems which rely on the principle that physicians should communicate suspected adverse effects to a neutral national agency have often failed because of underreporting.

An increasing number of British doctors are sending reports to the British Committee on the Safety of Medicines, but this may be an exception (Lawson and Wilson, 1974; WHO, 1972). Central agencies, however, whether national licensing authorities or supranational bodies will usually hesitate to inform physicians on possible adverse reactions to a drug before they are satisfied that there is a causal relationship: such satisfaction may require a large number of observations, i.e. considerable avoidable human suffering.

There is a good case for publishing in current medical journals any information on suspected adverse drug effects, even if it is not certain whether ill-effects observed were actually due to a drug (Editorial, 1978). Publication of such communications from physicians may induce other physicians to watch carefully the patients given a drug and may thus accelerate publication or collection of further information. Of course, there is a danger that overreporting of suspected adverse drug reactions might depreciate such information to such an extent that it is no longer read.

However, this point of oversaturation seems unlikely to be reached anywhere at present because physicians are not usually prolific writers, even of letters to journals. It is evidently *not* unfair for journal editors to publish isolated observations of suspected adverse drug reactions, while at the same time insisting that reports on alleged drug benefits be substantiated by statistically controlled methods (Editorial, 1978).

Failures to confirm claimed benefits from a drug, even in systematic studies, are 'negative results' and as such as not usually published. Consequently, practising physicians often may decide to use a drug because they are ill-informed on the benefit/risk ratio which tends to be lower than they imagine.

(3) Positive (higher benefit than assumed, fewer adverse effects than expected) or negative (less benefit than claimed; more adverse effects than anticipated) information on drugs may be available and even have been published in some journals, without reaching a prescriber's attention. This state of affairs probably occurs still more frequently than the absence of publication of relevant data. In as far as positive results are concerned, the danger of non-information is small since manufacturers (or importers) will diffuse any type of positive information on their products, however flimsy. This is unfortunately not so for negative results. No practising physician can be expected to read, or at least to scan more than one or two weekly, and perhaps additionally, one monthly, journal. Furthermore, though many younger phyisicians in highly developed countries now have some knowledge of English, besides their mother-tongue, no practising physician can be expected to read regularly a journal not published in his mother-tongue.

Much relevant published information on prescribed drugs of a negative character, therefore, escapes the attention of practising physicians in most countries. Editors of many large-circulation medical weeklies run an abstracting service to convey to their readers some of the information published elsewhere. For a great number of European medical weeklies these abstracting services, however, are quite inadequate and, furthermore, are rarely centred on drug effects.

Finally, it must be stated quite candidly that financially most medical journals depend heavily on the advertising of the drug industry. Wherever there is competition between different medical journals for a given market of practising physicians, the drug companies must be expected to use their financial influence in order to block the diffusion of information detrimental to the sales of their products: drug companies, after all, are not philanthropic organisations but, under most existing social systems, are compelled to make profits in order to survive. Any influence of manufacturers, importers or the trade on the distribution of information on drugs is obviously undesirable.

In developing countries, the situation is usually even worse. Physicians and other prescribers often cannot read regularly the current type of medical journals, and the drug companies have, for practical purposes, the monopoly of information, which they convey to prescribers by sometimes incredibly large numbers of representatives as well as by a strong hold on the contents of lists of (old and new) drugs which may be circulated to prescribers (Yudkin, 1978).

Several methods have been devised in a few highly developed countries for eliminating such influences. Monopolies of medical journals for large countries may be effective; if many physicians subscribe to the same journal, this journal may gain a position allowing it to resist pressures from advertisers, and even to impose some principles of advertising. Journals which have a virtual monopoly in their country, e.g. the *British Medical Journal* and *The Lancet* in Britain, are much freer than their counterparts in other countries to inform physicians on negative aspects of drugs according to the standards set by the editors of the journals. Though a dominant position gives some freedom of information to the editors of a journal, it does not make them altogether free from joint pressures by large groups or alliances of drug producers, unless the journal is financially viable even without any advertisements.

The second more effective way of informing prescribers on all aspects of drugs, without any risk of pressure by producers or distributors, is the production of journals dealing only with drug problems (with the understanding that other medical problems which bear less directly on industrial interests may be dealt with in those other journals which depend on pharmaceutical advertising). Such journals dealing only with drug problems do not carry any publicity and are sold to prescribers at a correspondingly higher price. Excellent and very successful examples of such journals are the American *Medical Letter*, the British *Drug and Therapeutics Bulletin*, the German *Arzneimittelbrief* or the (French) Swiss *Pharma-Flash*. Such journals are, for financial reasons, somewhat limited in their possibilities of covering all relevant drug news for prescribers (the most complete coverage among the journals cited being realised in the *Arzneimittelbrief*). Editing such a journal implies a considerable financial risk, which a journal editor may be capable of assuming or which may be shared by financially powerful organisations. Such an organisation can be (as in the case of the *Drug and Therapeutics*

Bulletin) a consumers' association. Recourse to other financially powerful organisations may be far more risky because these may be connected to the drug manufacturers, by links of which even the editor of an advertisement-free journal may not be aware.

There are even recent examples of apparently independent, advertisement-free drug information journals which are subsidised by one group of pharmaceutical manufacturers. To be valuable, advertisement-free drug journals must reach a certain circulation. They can, therefore, succeed only in countries with a large number of physicians of whom a sufficiently large fraction can be persuaded to subscribe to such a journal. The journals, of course, can extend their influence beyond national boundaries, but this will automatically increase their production costs, since presentations, proprietary names and prices of drugs may vary considerably from one state to another, even if both states use the same language. The attempt to found an advertisement-free journal for a small country, or in a language spoken only by a limited number of physicians, would be financially doomed in advance.

A third and most promising way for conveying unbiased drug information to all physicians is the production of advertisement-free drug journals by government authorities. The financial risks of such journals are knowingly borne by the taxpayer, who should also profit from the improved information of his physicians. It should, however, be borne in mind that the taxpayer, less directly, also pays for all information or misinformation on drugs which pharmaceutical manufacturers choose to convey to prescribers and consumers. In small countries, the burden of independent drug information journals on the taxpayers may appear too heavy, if a journal is to be produced entirely in the country: under these circumstances, government authorities would presumably be well-advised to enter into agreements with advertisement-free journals of other countries in order to use their materials. Government-issued drug information journals exist in Great Britain, Holland, Norway, Sweden and will, hopefully, be founded in many other countries in the near future.

(4) Prescribing physicians supplied with adequate information on merits and demerits of drugs may be either unwilling to or incapable of acting according to the information given to them.

Unwillingness to comply with recommendations based on the conclusions of controlled trials is fairly common. Many physicians fail to understand the statistical nature of their own recommendations: since the reaction of a given individual is, by its very nature, unpredictable, all use of drugs is based on statistical probabilities derived from studies on groups of human beings. This is a very simple statement which, to a greater or less extent, applies to all human activities: yet it may be very difficult to understand for members of a profession which still retain some of the privileges and types of action of infallible priests. More often, though to some extent realising the statistical nature of his recommendations, a physician will feel that he has observed benefit where controlled trials show none, or else that an adverse drug effect observed by others just does not occur in his patients. Though this feeling may correspond to the facts in isolated patient communities who have developed particular hereditary traits, it is unlikely to be justified within countries of a similar state of economic development and with a racially similar population. Though the response to certain drugs may differ in different individuals for genetic reasons, the likelihood that genetically similar individuals gather in certain communities is very small for most modern countries. Therefore, 'racial differences' complacently invoked by producers must be viewed with some suspicion.

Where not too frequent adverse drug effects are concerned, racial peculiarities of the inhabitants of the country in which such effects were first described are currently invoked by manufacturers and distributors of drugs in order to defend their continued sale in other countries. Thus American physicians had been warned, although not always successfully (*Journal Amer. Med. Assoc.*, 1968), against the danger of inducing aplastic anaemia by chloramphenicol in the early 1950s and yet, between 1965 and 1970, many manufacturers and distributors of chloramphenicol in Europe claimed that the occurrence of this adverse effect in North America was due to either particular racial features or to particular foods of the inhabitants of the North American continent: the drug was thus still promoted and used for a number of purposes when it should have been replaced by less dangerous drugs. This went on for about ten years, i.e. the time required to confirm that the incidence of aplastic anaemia after chloramphenicol in Europe did not differ from that on the American continent. Similar attitudes were usually taken in respect to the induction of subacute myelo-optic neuropathy (SMON) by the rather ineffective intestinal disinfectant clioquinol (Meade, 1975), and possibly by related compounds such as broxyquinoline.

Prescribers often are unable to use the information provided to them, either by lack of intelligence, or by absolute or relative overload with practical work not leaving time for required reading, or by linguistic inability to understand information provided in a foreign language, or finally by inadequate basic training in pharmacology and/or in medical therapeutics. A physician working in a small country may never obtain any unbiased drug information in his own language, while promotional material is nearly always translated into all languages. He may also fail to understand information provided in a foreign tongue. Such realistic drug information as is provided by the journals discussed above must, furthermore, by its very nature be short and couched in technical terms. Inadequate undergraduate training of physicians in pharmacology and medical therapeutics may result in an inability to understand condensed information. Furthermore, the authors contributing to such journals differ greatly in their ability to express information in simple and easily understood terms. The general medical and educational level of many practising physicians, furthermore, is such that they more easily retain and make use of spoken than of printed information. This is one of the reasons for the large-scale use of medical representatives by drug manufacturers. Unfortunately, those seeking to provide physicians with unbiased drug information have not so far tried to convey this information orally by suitable trained representatives.

There are thus many reasons why medical prescribers may be inadequately informed on what they prescribe and fewer reasons why they sometimes are adequately informed. The primary motivation of a prescribing physician for acquiring full information on the drugs he uses is, of course, his moral and legal responsibility to and for his patient.

Moral responsibility depends on ethical standards and may be difficult to improve in a system of medical care in which it carries no reward. As an incentive, reward may be replaced or complemented by punishment.

Legal responsibility may be defined as a liability for a prescriber for damage caused by his failure to heed information potentially available to him. In penal and civil malpractice cases, codes in different highly developed countries, however, differ widely in the reading requirements which they impose on doctors. While no one is primarily allowed to be uninformed about laws, doctors tend to be legally allowed to be uninformed on the contents of large numbers of medical publications. Furthermore, legal responsibility becomes a consideration of medical practice only when the attention of attorneys is drawn to possible malpractice, by individual patients, by patients' organisations or by advisory groups.

Thus, while it is an individual physician's responsibility to heed such information as he may obtain, it should be a political responsibility for licensing authorities to provide physicians with the most unbiased, most complete and readily understood information on drugs which they are allowed to prescribe. Legislators, as well as executive authorities concerned with public health, should assume the burden of this responsibility Public health authorities may resort to many different measures to ensure that physicians are correctly informed about drugs and to protect them against biased information.

On the negative side, public health authorities should strictly control all promotional activities of manufacturers, importers and distributors of drugs. Laws and regulations concerning the control of these promotional activities differ widely from country to country and in many apparently highly 'developed' countries prove to be quite 'underdeveloped'; while, on the other hand, the laws and the regulations (though not necessarily their enforcement) are sometimes quite overdeveloped in apparently underdeveloped countries.

Differences in legal, social and political systems may prevent attempts to unify legislation on the control of drug promotional activities in different countries. A strong case may, however, be made for the establishment of international recommendations on the aims to be pursued by such legislation. Such recommendations might show legislators what they should endeavour to do.

On the positive side, public health authorities can improve the information of prescribers on drugs by providing information which may, otherwise, remain inaccessible. Publishing drug journals is just one way of attempting to do this. Other media than print should, however, be used. Open or closed-circuit television, already extensively used in some countries for medical education in fields other than the use of drugs, could be increasingly utilised, and video-tapes may be distributed to physicians. Public health authorities should possess several rapid communication systems in order to inform about dangerous adverse effects or interactions, either newly discovered or suspected. In those countres in which representatives of manufacturers or importers are known to exert a major influence on doctors' prescribing habits, the state's public health authorities should attempt to control the number of representatives and the information conveyed by them. On the other hand, public health authorities of many countries would be well advised to consider setting up their own medical representative system.

At present, in many industrialised countries, public health

authorities fail to face their responsibility to contribute to full information of physicians and appear content to leave the drug scene to an open fight between a powerful industry and trade and a few well-intentioned individuals. This state of affairs is not in the long run compatible with citizens' justified expectations.

Use of Drugs by Health Workers not Fully Trained in Medicine

In most parts of the world, the number of physicians available to the population is far below the standards of the highly developed countries and far too small to permit that even the use of essential drugs (WHO, 1977) could be controlled by fully trained physicians. In most parts of the world, therefore, drugs are not prescribed, but are distributed, against payment or free of charge, by state-appointed health workers or self-appointed healers who are not fully trained in medicine, and may even subsist on information handed down from one generation to the next or from a non-medical master to his pupils. The problem of bringing information on drugs to these non-medical 'prescribers' is even more complicated than that of providing information to physicians.

Partly medically trained health workers or medical auxiliaries are called by different names, such as: *feldsher*, 'bare-foot doctor', 'health officer', *aide sanitaire*, *infirmier*, *fonctionnaire de centre de santé*, etc. in different countries: the extent of their training and of their power of decision differs widely. The partial medical training given to some of these groups of health workers hardly ever comprises a training in basic or in clinical pharmacology, though an attempt could be made to give the latter independently of the former (which depends on some training in physiology). It may, however, be extremely difficult to find or to train clinical pharmacologists prepared to teach their subject without any reference to basic processes. Furthermore, the grade of literacy of health workers may vary considerably. Medical field personnel may fluently read and write a national or international language (English, French, Russian or Chinese) in which they have been trained, but which may not be their mother-tongue; they may also be quite literate in their mother-tongue, but in no other language in which information is available. Furthermore, like many citizens of highly developed countries, even highly literate health workers may dread the effort of reading and, in the absence of a strong motivation, may therefore fail to use information provided for them. On the other hand, the reading or linguistic abilities of non-medical health workers may be so low that they can gain no effective information from printed material given to them. Providing adequate drug information to non-medically qualified health personnel appears to be one of the most difficult tasks of public authorities, responsible for controlling the work of these persons. To the best of my knowledge, none of the systems devised for this purpose has yet been shown to be reasonably successful. Experience gathered in many parts of the world allows one to draw up a catalogue of 'don'ts' which leaves authorities with few useful solutions, but should stimulate the imagination of planners and scientists in this field.

Some of the 'don'ts' may be summarised as follows.

(1) Never allow a health worker to distribute drugs on which he has not been informed beforehand. There is no point in providing him with the drugs and letting him have the information when his stocks are exhausted.

(2) Strictly limit the number of drugs available to non-medical distributors and try to ensure that no non-medical distributor is responsible for more than 20-50 drugs. Unlimited access to all drugs on a national list or even to all drugs on the list of essential drugs of WHO is likely to exceed the information-handling capacities of health workers without a full medical training.

(3) Never allow a change of brand name, package size, unit dose strength, colour or shape of the medicament or colour or shape of packages to occur without informing the health workers beforehand.

(4) Any direct contact between health workers and representatives of manufacturers or importers must be strictly prevented. By their lack of medical training and also by the fact that usually they receive low salaries, partially trained health workers are too easily subject to pressures which even physicians in highly developed countries sometimes resist only with great difficulty.

(5) Health workers should never be given information on drugs with long lists of indications, i.e. diseases, syndromes or symptoms against which a drug is more or less useful. Health workers should have a clear description of the effects of a drug and be given a very restrictive list of conditions under which these effects may be useful. They must be discouraged from making any therapeutic promises, but must also be given descriptions of drug effects which clearly distinguish between effects resulting in a possible cure,

effects which depend on long-term or life-long treatment and short-term symptomatic effects.

How then should non-medically trained health workers be informed on drugs? All information must be conveyed in a language which the recipient, the health worker, will completely understand. This means that in many countries such information will have to be prepared in more than one language, of which one could be a supranational international language, one a national language and several others vernacular languages (idioms) (Rougemont *et al.*, 1975; Belloncle *et al.*, 1980). Technical terms must be used only to the extent to which they are certain to be understood: particular skill may be required in transcribing technical into popular terms without losing precision. In many developing countries an international language is, generously, supposed to be known by all health workers who, in fact, can use this language in simple everyday commercial dealings but do not possess it sufficiently well to understand instructions. Under these conditions responsible health authorities may either prepare the information in a local language or attempt to ensure that health workers receive sufficient training in the international language to understand instructions. The easiest way of conveying information is of course the distribution of printed material, provided that great care is taken to avoid loss of the material by supplying it with special binders or folders which may be checked.

Since no drug should ever reach a prescriber, a distributor or a consumer (see Hermann *et al.*, 1978) without information on its use, extensive package inserts may appear a possible means for conveying that information. Unfortunately, the information required by these three categories of people is quite different in respect to its contents as well as to its language. Furthermore, over-information will usually result in complete disregard for all information provided. Finally, package inserts lose all possible impact whenever original packs are destroyed before the drugs are distributed without package inserts.

Difficulties about reading printed material have been discussed above, and printed information may have to be replaced by oral information. Again, the ideal way of transmitting oral information would be some type of phonetic record (tapes, records, etc.) but the use of such records depends on the availability of machinery with the sources of electricity required for their permanent and repeated use. Broadcasting may be used to convey information to health workers but, in the absence of recording, broadcasts on given topics must be repeated frequently in order to leave imprints in the memory of those concerned.

Training courses are often used for conveying information, but usually are not very successful with personnel of low grade literacy. Any success of lecture courses depends on notes taken by the participants or summaries distributed to them; both ways of recording information depend on literacy.

Finally and with similar reservations, public medical representatives with a higher grade of instruction, sent around by responsible health authorities, may be quite effective in conveying and distributing information, and their effectiveness may be reinforced by regular or irregular inspection tours of health authority physicians.

The most important problem, however, is the content of the information on drugs for health workers, not fully trained in medicine. These contents should, of course, be very different from those of drug information for physicians. First of all, health workers without medical training must be informed on the properties and effects of drugs but must also be informed on the features, causes and courses of diseases, illnesses or symptoms to be treated by these drugs. In order to simplify matters, one may be tempted to include into drug information sheets diagnostic criteria for diseases or symptoms to be treated (WHO, 1977). This procedure may be applicable to drugs used exclusively for treating one particular disease, i.e. a minority of the drugs which will be available on any limited national or international list.

Generally, however, a drug will be useful for treating more than one ailment, which may be a disease, an illness or a symptom. In that case, the drug information should contain a very restrictive list of indications; but health workers should be provided with particular information sheets on any one of these indications which, in turn, should include lists of all drugs that might be useful and, if possible, brief discussions of their respective merits. Any health worker should therefore possess separate files of information on symptoms and diseases on the one hand, and on therapeutic drugs on the other hand. The overall contents of drug information sheets for health workers may be similar to that of sheets for physicians, but the emphasis must be switched from theoretical to practical aspects (discussions on mechanisms of action should be limited to the information which is really useful to a non-medical prescriber). Furthermore, warnings or descriptions of adverse effects and interactions must be very clearly expressed in non-technical language. Still more than physicians, medical auxiliaries tend to overestimate possible benefits and to underestimate adverse effects of drugs! All descriptions should, furthermore, clearly indicate when a patient, showing a particular adverse effect, must be transferred to a health centre with a fully trained physician and how urgent such transfer is in a given set of conditions.

Finally, drug descriptions should carry indications of the size of stocks which non-medically trained health practitioners are recommended to keep at their disposal according to local needs.

Drug information for non-medically trained health officers may be prepared from internationally suggested drug information sheets, but there will probably not be a single instance in which the international text may simply be translated or transmitted without having been rewritten entirely according to the needs of a particular region (Rougemont *et al.*, 1975).

As stated above (see p. 105), non-medical health workers should be asked to use only a limited number of drugs. These drugs should be selected from 'standard' medicines known to physicians for at least 5 to 10 years. Problems due to unforeseen adverse effects or interactions may thus become less frequent. Yet, even with old drugs, warnings about newly discovered adverse effects may have to be transmitted to health workers. Again, all explanations must be 'translated', only essential information must be transmitted; and suggested withdrawals of drugs must be explained if they are to be enforced.

Healers who may be witch-doctors, traditional tribal physicians, religiously inspired health prophets (*marabout*), etc., nowadays use drugs originating from Western medicine which they will distribute themselves to patients, usually without disclosing the identity of the drug. Wherever this may be so, health authorities should try to let the self-appointed healers have full and understandable information on the drugs which they use. This information should be recorded and written in the same way as information for non-medically qualified health workers. Having the local healers informed on the drugs they use may be far more effective than prohibiting such use, because it will usually be very difficult to enforce prohibitions.

Most of the drugs which non-medically trained healers will use, however, will not belong to the Western therapeutic armamentarium but will be local traditional drugs of herbal or animal nature on which information usually cannot be transmitted to users, because it is just not available. The merits of proposals to revive or to sustain existing traditional medical systems in various countries cannot be discussed here. It should, however, be stressed that most traditional drugs are insufficiently standardised and that their beneficial or adverse effects and possible interactions, therefore, will vary considerably from one batch to the next, used by different practitioners of traditional medical systems.

If and where traditional drugs are to be used, they should first be carefully investigated and standardised. This requirement involves a tremendous amount of work by specialists who are usually not available. Information on traditional medicines, therefore, will usually be limited to information on adverse effects, the absence of beneficial effects or on interactions observed by chance – and such information can only be obtained if traditional healers or health practitioners, without full medical training, are not chased by the police, but receive a certain amount of official recognition.

Nurses

In developing countries, nurses often are the medical auxiliaries in charge of dispensaries or health centres. In that case they act as non-medically trained prescribers as discussed above.

In highly developed countries, nurses act as substitute prescribers under many different conditions. In many hospitals, nurses are authorised to distribute 'current need' medicaments, such as sleeping pills or laxatives. Outpatient clinic nurses often actually distribute drugs or prescriptions. Nurses working in the community are often consulted on drugs to be taken and actually prescribe 'drugs' which, by law, are not prescription drugs. Whenever nurses act as substitute prescribers, they should be informed on the drugs with which they deal to the same extent as are physicians. Nurses cannot be expected to read physicians' professional journals. Information on drugs must be relayed to them by other means, such as drug information sheets, small text-books and, wherever possible, articles in nurses' journals. Information given to nurses on non-prescription (over-the-counter) drugs should be more explicit than that given to the average consumer and could consist in the distribution of drug information sheets actually prepared for physicians. The training of nurses in basic pharmacology being usually still less adequate than that of physicians, there may be difficulties of understanding which, however, can be overcome.

Should nurses be thoroughly informed on prescription drugs? They are not allowed to distribute these drugs on their own authority and one might, therefore, argue that they do not need specific knowledge. Nurses do, however, play a role in the prescribing of drugs by physicians in many settings. They tend to be better informed than physicians on the patients' drug-taking which even under the most favourable conditions usually deviates considerably from the prescribed pattern (Latiolais and Berry, 1969; Sigstad *et al.*, 1972; Yudkin, 1978). Their more direct contact with patients allows them often to discover the occurrence of a known side effect or even to suspect a relationship between new symptoms or signs and the use of drugs. Finally, being charged with checking the patients' use of the drugs prescribed, they often discover overprescribing by a given physician or incompatibilities between different drugs prescribed. For all these reasons, there is a good case for requiring that nurses be informed, whenever possible, on all drugs prescribed by the physicians with whom they work. Given reasonable prescribing habits, i.e. a limited number of drugs used by each physician, this requirement can presumably be fulfilled. Unfortunately, few attempts are made to do so.

Consumers

Consumers, on the one hand, are those who make the final decision to use or not to use a drug (unless it is injected into them by medical personnel). On the other hand, the consumer is the one who may personally suffer the adverse effects or adverse interactions of drugs, and such suffering may or may not be compensated by symptomatic or therapeutic benefit. Consumers are therefore entitled to the fullest possible information on drugs which they use on their own initiative or because they have been advised to do so by medical personnel.

No other information in the whole chain, unfortunately, is as difficult as that for consumers, mainly because they vary enormously in their literacy, their general education, their medical and their biological knowledge. Therefore, when information is formulated for consumers, correct interpretation of medical, pharmaceutical or biological terms used can never be taken for granted, not even in highly developed countries.

Consumers also differ greatly in their understanding of their own mother-tongue, of accepted national languages and of more or less international idioms. Finally, there are classes of consumers such as children or, as a matter of fact, a fraction of the aged population of any country, who are constitutionally incapable of understanding information on drug effects which may be given to them. Someone else must take the responsibility for their drug-taking, even if other responsibilities can still be assumed by these persons. Consumers, presumably, should be given some general information on the availability, the uses and the dangers of drugs. This will be discussed below.

In as far as specific information about a drug which somebody wants to take, or is told to take, is concerned, consumers' information must be handled differently for over-the-counter drugs and for prescription drugs.

Over-the-counter drugs are bought and taken on the consumer's own initiative; the choice of the drug may be guided by some general knowledge but, more often, is inspired by advice given to potential consumers by publicity or, sometimes, by specific advice given by pharmacists, neighbours, relatives or friends. Self-medication with manufactured, well-characterised drugs began to play a big social and economical role towards the end of the 19th century and attained its all-time maximal extent towards 1920. By this time about 80 to 90 per cent of all drugs sold were sold without actual medical advice (*Conseil de l'Europe*, 1975). Between 1920 and 1960, the percentage fraction of over-the-counter drugs in total drug sales, expressed as units or as value, has consistently declined but, in most countries, has remained fairly constant since approximately 1960. Absolute sales of over-the-counter drugs in different highly developed countries, however, have tended to stabilise already since approximately 1950. This means that the number of people purchasing over-the-counter drugs and the amount of drugs taken by these people presumably has remained fairly constant during the last 30 years with a possible downward trend since 1975 or 1976 in a few countries. Many people thus appear to feel that they need some drugs and that these drugs help them. This may not be so; expert opinion on the medical value of self-medication is divided (*Conseil de l'Europe*, 1975).

Furthermore, there is little doubt that a fraction of the use of over-the-counter drugs represents drug dependence of different grades of severity and medical importance. This applies to hypnotics (for which, however, a prescription is usually required, though there are always some exceptions readily discovered by addicts), and also to such generally used drugs as laxatives, cough medicines and minor analgesics. The policy of legislators and licensing authorities concerning over-the-counter drugs will, therefore, to some extent determine the nature of drug dependencies and the number of drug-dependent subjects in a country.

Decisions on the number of drugs allowed to be sold over-the-counter and the selection of such drugs, therefore, are amongst the most difficult tasks of legislators and licensing authorities. If they are generous, they will increase the sales of over-the-counter drugs, the number of people suffering from adverse effects and the number of addicts to these drugs. If, on the other hand, they are too restrictive, they will encourage people, unwilling to seek medical advice, to resort to other types of medical care, such as mystical therapeutic measures which may be innocent, but also to traditional old-time medicines which may actually represent a growing danger in highly developed countries.

The realisation that many synthetic medicaments, even among those administered for over-the-counter sales, may have dangerous adverse effects has in recent years led to an increased consumption of medicinal herbs, usually taken as teas but also sometimes added to food. Such herbs are often sold to the public by persons who, in contrast to their predecessors a century ago, are neither familiar with the botanical characteristics of such herbs, nor with methods of collecting and of storing them.

Even when traditional precautions are well-known and applied, herbal medicines may be dangerous, because their composition and content of pharmacologically active substances may be extremely variable. Moreover, the toxicology of traditional herbal medicaments is usually completely unknown. For other over-the-counter medicaments, there is usually a fairly large body of information on toxic effects in experimental animals and on adverse effects in man. For medicinal herbs, usually, even the lethal dose in animals is unknown and possible toxic effects of long-term use in animals or in man have never been investigated. Replacing over-the-counter drugs by herbal medicine, therefore, is tantamount to replacing known and partially avoidable risks by completely unknown dangers.

In developing countries, on the other hand, ancestral knowledge of traditional herbal medicines may still be more or less current, sometimes even despite long periods of colonial domination. Such ancestral knowledge may avoid acute poisoning, but practically never comprises any information on potential long-term toxic effects. None the less, governments of developing countries sometimes choose to encourage the use of traditional herbal medicines in order to avoid the spending of scarce public funds on expensive and often dangerous foreign drugs.

Information which leads to the selection of one rather than another over-the-counter drug, if it is not provided by professionals like pharmacists or nurses, or even druggists, usually originates from producers' publicity displayed either in drug-store windows, in newspapers or, where this is still legal, on radio or television. In most countries, this type of publicity partially or totally escapes the control of licensing authorities. In some countries, it is counterbalanced to some extent by the activity of consumers' associations. Though sometimes powerful, these associations, however, never have financial means comparable to those of drug producers and, therefore, have less influence on the actual purchase and taking of drugs, the effect of publicity being by and large proportional to the amounts of money spent on it (Fern, 1975; Nord, 1976).

It is evident that all information on drugs carried by publicity should be strictly controlled by public health authorities, preferably by the officials engaged in the licensing of drugs. Publicity for over-the-counter drugs is usually made for one brand of a drug sold under a proprietary name. It is a truism to state that any effective control of the use of over-the-counter drugs requires that the active ingredients of such drugs should be stated everywhere in the publicity and on packages by giving their non-proprietary (generic) names. Such use of generic names, established by law and enforced, is a prerequisite for any effective prevention of economic abuse of the over-the-counter drug market. Unfortunately, the use of non-proprietary names for such drugs is not legally required and enforced in all countries.

Specific information on a drug, purchased without medical prescription, is usually provided in package inserts. Again, the contents of such package inserts vary widely from drug to drug, from producer to producer, from country to country: even package inserts for the same drug sold in different countries by the same company vary considerably, and not necessarily in order to make them suit local public health needs (Herxheimer, 1974; Yudkin, 1978).

It is evident that package inserts should be understandable to a huge majority of prospective consumers. They should, therefore, be written in clear popular language and should contain no statements which might be misunderstood. In countries with more than one language, they must be multilingual; the problems of reading and understanding package inserts in countries with large fractions of illiterate citizens have not been resolved. It is evident that the contents of package inserts should be carefully checked and controlled by health authorities and such a control should be compulsory;

unfortunately, this is generally not so. Measures for ensuring strict control of the contents of package inserts of all drugs sold without prescription, and the publication of precise rules for the contents of such inserts are therefore urgent tasks for public health authorities, as well as legislators of all countries. A good case can be made for uniform, state-produced package inserts for the most widely used over-the-counter drugs. Again, since most of the drugs sold over the counter in large amounts are the same in many countries, it would be advisable to draw up international standard package inserts for these drugs (*Ad hoc* Working Group, 1977).

Such inserts could be modified by local health authorities in countries in which particular warnings or recommendations must be added. Package inserts written for the layman and understandable to the layman with the lowest cultural standards must of course never be mixed up with drug information leaflets written for physicians or other health professionals. Health authorities in many countries will find it difficult to write package inserts on the basis of such international drug information leaflets.

The contents of the package insert for an over-the-counter drug can easily be delimited (Hermann *et al.*, 1978). The package insert should state the non-proprietary name of the drug and the nature of its main effect ('eliminates pain for 3-5 hours by an action on the brain'; 'will induce one or several bowel movements or diarrhoea 8-10 hours after taking, by irritating the colon'; 'will prevent vitamin deficiency during pregnancy'; etc.); the usual dose and recommended mode of administration; the maximal allowed dose, both for a single administration and for a 24-hour period; a statement whether the drug can be used in children and, if so, at what dose levels for what body weight or age; a statement whether the drug can be used in elderly people and, if so, at what dose levels; warnings concerning possible interactions or incompatibility, as well as a general warning not to use the drug simultaneously with any medicament prescribed by a physician without seeking the physician's advice; and a description of the main side effects which might occur, with some statement about their frequency and precise instructions to the consumer on the action to be taken if one of the side effects described occurs ('immediately stop taking the drug; no other action required'; 'immediately consult a doctor'; 'stop taking the drug and consult your doctor within the next three days'; etc.).

A package insert should not contain a list of indications for the use of a given drug; should not enumerate all possible side effects that have ever been suspected to be caused by the drug; and should not discuss mechanisms of action in great detail. A package insert must always be short; its total length should never exceed two type-written pages.

Wherever the sale of over-the-counter drugs can be restricted to pharmacists, the pharmacist should be held responsible for giving patients appropriate warnings against possible side effects and instructions what to do about them. He should, of course, give patients detailed information on how and when to take a drug.

In the usual physician-patient relationship, the physician only tells the patient how and when to take a drug, and what to avoid while taking the drug, but quite often fails to inform him on the purpose of a prescription and on the effects expected. Patients, however, want to have this information (Mattar *et al.*, 1975; Joyce, 1961); they usually obtain it, partially, and in a very unsatisfactory manner, by reading the package inserts given them with the prescription drugs (Joubert and Lasagna, 1975) which, in most countries, are not really designed for informing patients. Package inserts for drugs manufactured in Europe are often just short summaries of more extensive standard information sheets designed for physicians.

Unfortunately, package inserts are also often used by physicians as an easily available summary of the more explicit standard information sheet. Package inserts of American medicaments, even if manufactured and distributed in Europe, on the other hand, usually are extremely complete information sheets written for physicians and contain an enormous amount of information on adverse effects, interactions, etc., often presented in very small print and practically unreadable. Neither the European nor the American type of package insert for most prescription medicines is really useful for patients.

Prescription drugs are, though, sold to consumers, i.e. patients in most countries, and not to doctors. Package inserts (Hermann *et al.*, 1978) should, therefore, be designed in such a manner that they give the patient some practical information which, in principle, should recall information received from his physician. The package insert for a prescription drug may contain a brief description of the effects and the mode of action of a drug; in no case should it contain a list of indications. It should indicate the recommended way of taking a drug, but contain a statement that this may be modified by the prescribing physician for particular purposes. Doses or the possibility of using a drug in children or in old people should not be discussed in this type of package insert.

The main adverse effects should be enumerated with instructions for the patient on what to do, but there should be a statement that other side effects might occur and that the prescribing physician will tell the patient about these. Interactions may or may not be enumerated but, again, there should be a statement that the physician, for particular reasons, might prescribe a given drug with other drugs with which it interacts. All this information will be helpful for the patient, but will be of value only if the prescribing physician has taken care to inform his patient on the purpose of the drug.

Of course, in the case of drugs used for common conditions or symptoms, prescribers may prepare written or printed information sheets for patients, which may replace oral instructions if and when the prescriber is sure that the written information will be understood. Wherever a patient is informed in writing on effects and possible adverse effects of a drug, there should be a statement encouraging him to ask his doctor about everything which he may want to know (Herxheimer, 1976) or did not understand. Successful drug therapy requires the patient's full collaboration and full collaboration is difficult to obtain in the absence of full information. On the other hand, being compelled to inform the patient in clear and simple words on the purpose of any drug prescription may prove extremely useful for prescribers and their rational use of medicaments.

Legislators and Policy-makers

Legislators and policy-makers interested in drafting bills or devising subsidiary legislation concerning drugs and public health should be informed not only on financial and economic aspects of the use of drugs but also on the medical and social role of groups of drugs used in the treatment or prevention of groups of symptoms or diseases. Ideally, legislators and policy-makers in the drug field should have as much training and information on drugs as prescribing physicians; in practice, this requirement can probably never be met.

Even if legislators and policy-makers are originally medically trained, their many other duties and needs for information often deprive them of the possibility of keeping abreast with progress and changes in the use of medicaments. Policy-makers and legislators, and also non-medically trained health officials, therefore need books and reviews, which unfortunately at present are rarely if ever available even in the most current languages. Many books have been published on general aspects of the use and the abuse of drugs, the organisation of the pharmaceutical industry or drug legislation. Even if they can gather some information from such books, legislators, policy-makers and officials would more specifically need two other types of book: firstly, a textbook on drug therapy for non-professionals, describing the use of drugs for people who are professionals in the fields of health and politics – such a book should be easy to read, relatively short and provide many references; secondly, an alphabetically arranged drug encyclopaedia, in which they can rapidly find information on the main features of a particular drug which may become important for legislative or political aspects of the drug markets at a given time. Books like the drug lists published by Pradal (1974) which, in fact, are written for consumers, might prove useful in this respect.

Again, there would be a good case for trying to produce similar books written specifically for the purposes of policy-makers and officials and containing statements about medical aspects, preventive and therapeutic, as well as economics, patent status and producers of major drugs. One might envisage a kind of Merck Index (Windholz *et al.*, 1976) for legislators, health officials and politicians, as well as people commercially interested in drugs. The publication of journals on the use of drugs suitable for political and administrative readers might also be considered.

Education in the Field of Drugs and their Effects

The efficacy of information on progress and change depends, of course, on the primary education received by the person to be informed. This statement applies to general education, as well as to specific education in the fields of pharmacology, the use of medicaments, and the effects of toxic agents. Information, on the other hand, is always conveyed at a certain level of previous training. While it is relatively easy to instruct groups of people whose previous training is similar, it is always difficult to inform people with very different educational backgrounds and with very different specific knowledge. One might, therefore, strive to ensure a fairly uniform and as extensive as possible education of professionals in the fields of pharmacology and of toxicology, but some attempts should also be made to provide and to maintain a certain education in the drug field in the general public, i.e. among consumers of drugs.

Physicians

The statement that the fraction of the medical curriculum devoted to training in pharmacology, toxicology and drug therapy is far too small when compared to the amount of time which practising physicians spend on selecting, prescribing and evaluating drugs remains true, though some progress has been made during the last 30 years. In most highly developed countries, medical schools do not actually train doctors, but provide only basic care training in medicine, which is subsequently completed by specialised training in one of the many medical professions. Systematic investigations, on the nature and the quantity of knowledge in pharmacology and toxicology which is or should be used in medical practice, unfortunately have not been made. The material presented in the medical curriculum, therefore, everywhere is determined to a large extent by traditions and assumed needs, rather than by actually measured needs.

Even though training in the drug field during the medical school years may approach adequacy, it is often inadequate during the post-medical school years when future doctors obtain their specialist's training. Training courses for specialists usually include far too little pharmacological information for practical purposes. The field which, therefore, should be developed in the education of physicians is presumably postgraduate teaching in pharmacology, toxicology and drug therapy during the years of specialisation, but also for physicians actually engaged in the practice of medicine.

Within medical schools, pharmacology in many countries is at present taught in two separate courses: a course on basic pharmacology given before or during the first year of clinical training, while a course on drug therapy is given towards the end of the clinical training. This teaching has considerably improved the pharmacological knowledge possessed by physicians, at least during the immediate postgraduate years. (This statement is an impression of a teacher in the field but, unfortunately, not the result of a systematic investigation.)

Health Workers not Trained in Medicine

This group of people, extremely important for the medical care of a large fraction of mankind, usually has received no basic education in pharmacology, toxicology and drug therapy. Information of such health workers on drugs would be greatly facilitated, and many mistakes could presumably be avoided, if a basic course in pharmacology and in toxicology could be included in whatever formal training they receive before being assigned to their duties. Devising such courses would be an interesting and important task for pharmacologists who are thoroughly familiar with the conditions of the country for which health workers are being trained.

Nurses

The important role of nurses in the distribution of drugs to consumers has been outlined above. Unfortunately, basic education in pharmacology is not provided in all professional nursing schools. A course in pharmacology and in the practical use of drugs (as well as some information on toxicology) should be included into the curriculum of all such schools and might prove more important than extensive instruction in the more fundamental fields of medical research which is usually included in the training of nurses.

Consumers

Educating potential or actual consumers of drugs, i.e. conveying to them information on the general limitations of the usefulness of drugs, on their possible adverse effects and interactions, as well as on their therapeutic merits, appears to be an enormous task. As a general rule, opinions on medical matters, in the public at large, faithfully reflect the officially accepted medical opinions of a bygone age, usually 30-50 years ago. In the less-developed countries the public opinion on medical matters may reflect still older notions. Education of the public in the drug field would presumably be much easier if it were a problem of educating people in matters on which they have no idea whatever. Unfortunately, in practice, education of the public on drugs implies eradication of widely held erroneous beliefs in favour of some basic knowledge.

Education of the public at large, i.e. of people engaged in many different walks of life, cannot consist in the organisation of courses, lectures or other traditional educational programmes. (Such information on human biology which is given in schools could presumably be complemented by information on the effects of drugs and toxic agents. This requirement will, of course, entail the need for some pharmacological education of teachers at various levels which might be quite difficult to organise at present.) Education of the public at large can only consist of repeated short and easily understood presentations in the mass media — the printed word, radio and television. Many media now actually run features or columns on medical matters which are often devoted to pharmacological problems. Unfortunately, the quality of the information conveyed in this way is very variable. Ways to improve this situation will have to be sought in the near future, but have not yet been devised.

Legislators and Policy-makers

The education of this group of people in the drug field presents problems as fundamental as those encountered with the general public, though slightly less complicated because the general level of education of this group is probably higher than that of the average citizen.

Responsibilities

Drugs can provide medical preventive as well as therapeutic benefits, but they create major problems too, by entailing morbidity, expenditure and social problems. Informing and educating about drugs are therefore major responsibilities which, everywhere in the world, should be assumed by governments and public health authorities.

References

Ad hoc Working Group (1977). Minimum information for sensible use of self-prescribed medicines. An international consensus. *Lancet 2*, 1017-19

Belloncle, G., Balique, H., Rougemont, A. and Ranque, P. (1980). Vernacular literacy produces good health workers. *World Health Forum 1*, 67-71

Conseil de l'Europe, Comité Européen de Santé Publique (1975). *L'abus des médicaments*, Rapport d'un groupe de travail (1972-1973), Strasbourg

Davies, D.M. (1977). Epidemiology. In Davies, D.M. (Ed.), *Textbook of Adverse Drug Reactions*, Oxford, Oxford University Press, 73-7

Editorial (1978). Communicating adverse drug reactions. *Lancet 1*, 133

Fern, M.A. (1975). Advertising. In Smith, M.C. (Ed.), *Principles of Pharmaceutical Marketing* (2nd Edn.), Lea and Febiger, Philadelphia, 292-313

Gardner, P. and Watson, L.J. (1970). Adverse drug reactions: a pharmacist-based monitoring system. *Clin. Pharmacol. Ther. 11*, 802-8

Hermann, F., Herxheimer, A. and Lionel, N.D.W. (1978). Package inserts for prescribed medicines: what minimum information do patients need? *Brit. Med. J. 2*, 1132-5

Herxheimer, A. (1979). Drug information: is there a need for international uniformity? *Drugs 8*, 321-9

—— (1976). Sharing the responsibility for treatment. How can the doctor help the patient? *Lancet 2*, 1294, 1976

Herxheimer, A. and Lionel, N.D.W. (1978). Minimum information needed by prescribers. *Brit. Med. J. 2*, 1129-32

Hollister, L.E. (1979). Drug product information: sensible disclosure of clinically important facts. *Drugs 7*, 414-18

Joubert, P. and Lasagna, L. (1975). Patient package insert. I. Nature, notions and needs. *Clin. Pharmacol. Ther. 18*, 507-12

Journal of the American Medical Association (1968). A report of a US Senate investigation. *J. Amer. Med. Ass. 203*, 11, News page 54

Joyce, C.R.B. (1961). Patient co-operation and the sensitivity of clinical trials. *J. Chron. Dis. 15*, 1025-33

Latiolais, C.J. and Berry, C.C. (1969). Misuse of prescription medicaments by outpatients. *Drug Intelligence and Clin. Pharmacy 3*, 270-7

Lawson, D.H. and Wilson, G.M. (1974). Detecting adverse drug reactions. *Brit. J. Hospital Med. 12*, 790-6

Mattar, M.E., Markello, J. and Yaffe, S.J. (1975). Inadequacies in the pharmacological management of ambulatory children. *J. Pediatrics 87*, 137-41

Meade, T.W. (1975). Subacute myelo-optic neuropathy and clioquinol. An epidemiological case-history for diagnosis. *Brit. J. Preventive and Social Med. 29*, 157-69

Nord, D. (1976). *Arzneimittelkonsum in der Bundesrepublik Deutschland*, Ferdinand Enke-Verlag, Stuttgart, 53-74

Pradal, H. (1974). *Guide des médicaments les plus courants* (3rd Edn.), Editions du Seuil, Paris

Rougemont, A., Balique, H., Boisson, M.E. and Péné, P. (1975). Une zone pilote d'enseignement et de recherche en épidémilogie, médicine et santé tropicales dans la région de Bamako, République du Mali. 2ème Réunion scientifique conjointe franco-britannique d'Epidémiologie et de Médicine sociale, Rennes, 24-26 juillet

Sigstad, H., Eivindson, A. and Hauge, I.J. (1972). Medikamenten forbruk i hjemmene. Tidsskrift Norske Laegeforening, *34*: 2319-23

WHO (1972). International drug monitoring: the role of national centres. *Technical Report Series 498*, Geneva

WHO (1977). The selection of essential drugs (report of a WHO Expert committee). *Technical Report Series 615*

Windholz, M., Budavari, S., Stroumtsos, L.Y. and Fertig, M.N. (Eds.) (1976). *The Merck Index. An Encyclopedia of Chemicals and Drugs* (9th Edn.), Rahway NJ, Merck and Co., Inc

Yudkin, J.S. (1978). Provision of medicines in a developing country. *Lancet 1*, 810-12

6 FACTORS AFFECTING INDIVIDUAL USE OF MEDICINES

Richard Blum, with Kevin Kreitman

Introduction

In this chapter, we examine immediate and proximate non-illness factors which influence the consumption of medicines by consumers. By 'immediate and proximate' are meant those variables with a direct and personal impact on the habits and decisions of the medicine user, as for example, prescriptions given to him by a doctor, drug information offered by the mass media, folk practices learned within the family, or psychological states which prompt a decision to purchase a compound. Excluded from consideration here are those variables, the diffuse impact of which is much the same for all persons in a biosocial class, region, geographical area or residence locale. Examples are the availability of one or another medicine, because of importation or manufacturing capacities in a nation, access to health services as a function of health care resources availability or the nature of professional criteria by which it is judged that one or another drug is appropriate for a diagnosed complaint. Excluded here as throughout this book, are pharmacotherapeutic and epidemiological considerations which describe appropriate and/or actual uses of medicines on the basis of disease and pertinent treatments.

In most modern nations, one will find both variation and constancy in the patterns of medicine use and in the belief and personal action systems which underlie these. For the most part, these variations will probably reflect the differential operation of factors which differentially distribute many beliefs and habits, not just those in the health arena. In the social sciences, these factors are, as gross categories, typically found to vary according to cultural heritage, socio-economic class, ideology, education, vocation, sex, age, residence (rural-urban) neighbourhood, family structure, individual attitudes and personality. In a typical modern nation there will be a number of population subgroups whose use of medicines can be successfully 'typed' according to these biosocial characteristics. There will be situations in which subgroup membership, however varied as defined by classifying features, may not predict variations in the use of medicines. An illustration would be a measles or smallpox threat which, in a nation effectively organised for public health, would lead to prophylactic injections for all the population, or, alternatively a nation so poor or isolated that no one has access to, say, gamma globulin in spite of the risk of a massive hepatitis outbreak.

With regard to the use of medicines, one of the most important features operating with respect to compliance to prescription recommendations and influences, will be the physician. Physician-related variables affecting consumer behaviour begin with the presence, absence or use of access to medical care, and extend to doctors' competence, attitudes toward prescribing, and behaviour with patients, for example, the extent to which they give clear and careful information and are attentive to patients' needs and questions. These aspects of doctors' behaviour are by no means constant, but vary with cultural milieu, age, education, practice characteristics, attitudes and personality, for example. Thus we see that social and psychological influences can affect consumer drug use indirectly, operating through the doctor, as well as directly in the person of the consumer himself.

In research on the role of non-illness factors which affect the use of medicines, it is generally necessary to control for illness; otherwise, this can certainly be overriding, obscuring the impact of other variables. Such experimental control should not, however, be mistaken for an actual separation in fact of social and individual factors from disease status, for disease, its diagnosis and its treatment 'career' are each influenced by environmental and personal circumstances. The result is that one may find some aspects of pathology and its treatment are associated with the very same social and personal influences which affect those belief systems or family habits which, in turn, account for the use of medicines when, among groups, disease status is experimentally controlled.

An example of the above would be, in a poor rural region, widespread infant gastrointestinal disorder, arising out of the inadequate sanitation, nutrition, medical care and self-care knowledge. Poverty and ignorance will be associated with both disease prevalence and folk treatment efforts, which rely (let us say) on herbals and magic rather than efficacious prevention and intervention. As another example, consider that hypochrondriacal anxiety state in a patient leading to a diagnosis of neurosis. The anxiety accounts not only for the diagnosis but is instrumental in the patient's self-prescribing large amounts of aspirin and alcohol and, at the same time, being prescribed tranquillisers. Such examples are commonplace. What is to be kept in mind is that the relationship between environmental, cultural, pathological and pharmacological variables is usually one of complex interdependence.

Existing Studies

Although sophisticated research, be that found in epidemiology, cultural medicine or medical psychology, does demonstrate the complex multi-determined nature of events leading to the use of medicine, such studies are few and far between. In the preparation of this chapter, we conducted a literature search utilising the computerised files of the US National Library of Medicine, the conventional abstract and reference volumes in medicine and the social sciences, and routine bibliographical tracking from citation to citation. Whilst that search took us over several thousand titles, there were remarkably few pertinent to the focus of this chapter. Most of the pertinent extant drug research bears on the self-administration of the illegal or sometimes socially disruptive psychoactive drugs (alcohol, heroin, cannabis, etc.). All of these drugs do have medical applications. Such 'drug abuse' literature offers convincing profound demonstrations of the critical nature of non-medical variables as determinants of drug use. Insofar as that literature contains data bearing on the self-administration of illicit psychoactives for pain relief or enhancement of feelings of well-being, it also calls attention to fundamental semantic and philosophical problems in the definition of health.

In this chapter as in this book, we exclude psychoactive drug 'abuse' from our purview. In doing so, the reader is denied that literature review, which most easily and powerfully demonstrates that how people view and what they do with pharmaceutical and folk medical compounds has much to do with their social circumstances, their aspirations, their feelings, their personalities, and very little to do with conventionally diagnosed illness and ordinary medical practice. Were the scientific literature more adequate as to the use of drugs within more typical healing systems, i.e. within those prosaic definitions of health which are promulgated by health authorities, the power of social and personal influences co-varying with disease in determining patterns of medicine use could be stated with some accuracy. Lacking these studies, as this chapter shows, one is reduced to the identification of a few simple variables which have been found, in limited settings and populations, to affect patient/consumer use of medicines.

Even the simplest of descriptive information is missing or inadequate. We had presumed that most nations would have available statistics on the per capita consumption of prescription and OTC compounds, their cost to manufacturers, health systems and consumers, and the correlations between at least major compounds' use and (diagnosed) disease prevalence. This is not so. One might also assume, given the billions of dollars spent worldwide in drug advertising, that there would be an ample literature detailing the effects of mass media information on drugs to consumers. To the contrary, we could find almost no studies in this area. A major reason is the belief in the pharmaceutical industry that such information is commercially sensitive and should therefore be kept secret. Prescriptions certainly account for much medicine that consumers, as patients, use. We had expected to find a scientific literature replete with studies on psychosocial variables affecting doctors' diagnostic, prescribing, and patient interactive processes. A few excellent studies do exist; but, for the most part, the study of prescribing as a psychological process is *terra incognita*.

The kind of health delivery system in which a patient/consumer is immersed, be that *laissez-faire*, private insurance, Western or Eastern socialist, or Chinese or Iranian rural paramedical, must certainly dictate some of the variation in the use of medicines. When, within a country, several such systems co-exist (as in the US), there is great opportunity to study within and between system variations on kind and manner of drug use and of related patient attitudes and knowledge. That opportunity has not been employed. Perhaps all of us handle the aspirations for and definition of health in very personal ways, these linked to family values, personal ideals, work roles, educational exposure and the like, yet there is only a beginning literature — some of it fine, indeed — on how personal conceptions of health are linked to the choice of remedies. Similarly, the range of substances available and used for healing in the home (be that palliative or restorative) is immense, from bats' wings and toads' eyes to teas, intoxicants and herbs by the hundreds. What is the everyday armamentarium of mothers, witches and wise women across a range of cultures; what does anthropology or pharmacognosy tell us? Not much more than Dioscorides did and certainly not, with very few exceptions, with the refinement of saying who, when and where.

Either for knowledge for its own sake, or for the practical purposes of knowing who uses what, when, so that one may estimate whether that use measured against some beneficial criteria might be altered, it would be wise to have the missing information at hand. It is not. For that reason, we offer our most telling conclusion first; our ignorance worldwide is great. If we are to improve the economic and health status of consumers, using specified beneficial criteria, we must learn more about their current use of medicines and the forces affecting that use and its outcomes.

Minimal Statistics

Consumption of both prescribed and non-prescription (OTC) pharmaceutical products is prevalent and widespread, particularly in technically advanced populations. Although accurate drug utilisation statistics are generally unavailable, Christopher and Crooks (1974) offer estimates. Prescriptions filled by chemists in England and Wales fluctuated between 188-212 million per year from 1949 to 1964. In 1970, on the average, each general practitioner in the UK wrote just over 12,900 prescriptions (Malleson, 1973). Inspection of annual data suggests that rates of prescribing continue to rise, even though there are fluctuations; compare 205.5 million prescriptions in England and Wales in 1963 with 246.2 in 1969, 266.5 in 1971 and 284.1 in 1973.

In Sweden, the National Board of Health reported a total of 20.9 million prescriptions in 1954 and a sharp increase to 38.1 million in 1968, again levelling off by 1970. According to United States estimates 2,000 million prescriptions were dispensed in 1970, a 50 per cent increase over the previous decade. Most of these (in 1975, 1.4 billion) are new drug orders, i.e. not repeat prescriptions. In the US in 1973, out-of-pocket prescription costs averaged about 24 dollars per person. The total national expenditure on drugs in France, adjusted for inflation, rose 170 per cent between 1959 and 1972. In the United States, over-the-counter (OTC) sales were $4.5 billion in 1976 including all products (cosmetic and dental) for which health claims were made.

Consumers and Medicines

Self-Medication

Rates of use of non-prescription compounds vary with the expected 'typical' biosocial characteristics and will, therefore, be shown to differ among studies sampling different populations. Differences by country have been shown by Herxheimer (1977); Great Britain, Canada and the US show greater non-prescription than prescription drug use; France, Yugoslavia and Argentina show the reverse. Overall, Americans take more drugs, prescribed and OTC (over-the-counter, not prescribed) than do Europeans. Of those Americans taking medicines, about half use OTCs alone or in addition to prescription substances.

In a longitudinal panel study in the UK, Knapp and Knapp (1962) reported that over 60 per cent of the illnesses occurring in the households studied were treated with non-prescribed drugs only. An average of 17 non-prescription drugs (including non-ingestibles such as skin creams) were on hand per household at the beginning of the study, compared with five prescribed drugs. An average of 8.5 OTC and 5.2 prescription drugs were procured per household during the 30-week study period. Though upper-class homes contained more drugs, the OTC to prescription drug ratio remained the same. Roney and Hall (in Johnson, 1976) found that households in California purchased an average of one OTC substance over a two-week period, with an average 24 such compounds on hand in the home. In an English study (Dunnell and Cartwright, 1972) 99 per cent of the homes surveyed had one or more medicines in it, an average of 3.0 prescribed and 7.3 non-prescribed. They found no significant difference in medicine use by social class but middle-class homes tended to have more OTC medicines. Even though over half the adults in the study reported that their health was good or excellent, most reported having experienced some symptoms of illness in the previous two-week period, and over half used some medicine during that time. OTCs accounted for two-thirds of the drug use, most often aspirin and analgesics, which were taken by 41 per cent of the adults; digestive remedies were used by 25 per cent. In a British study, Wadsworth *et al.* (1971) reported a similar distribution. Two-thirds of the medicines used by the population were not prescribed by a physician.

A World Health Organisation medical care utilisation study (Matthews and Feather, 1976) of 15,000 persons in Canada found that prescribed and non-prescribed medication had been used by over 50 per cent of the study population in the preceding 48 hours; non-prescribed medicines accounted for over half of this use.

In addition to the descriptive question, how much non-prescription drug use occurs (this was answered for Western countries by the foregoing studies), there are two other general queries addressed in the literature. One asks what kinds of people employ OTC drugs and under what circumstances does such use occur; the other asks essentially whether or not widespread OTC use is a good or bad thing. The latter value judgement is ordinarily transformed – and perhaps attenuated – by asking whether self-treatment is appropriate, that is, are OTCs generally employed for conditions which require relief but do not necessitate medical attention? The alternative is that self-medication occurs as a substitute for medical care (less desirable to the extent that medical care is the more efficacious).

With regard to OTC-user characteristics and circumstances, the following is a summary. Self-medication varies with symptoms and sex; fever, headache, sore throat and digestive problems are more likely to be self-medicated than other symptoms (Herxheimer, 1977; Johnson *et al.*, 1976). Women are more likely than men to self-medicate and to buy OTC drugs (Herxheimer, 1977; Bush and Rabin, 1976; Dunnell and Cartwright, 1972). Whites, people visiting primary care specialists, people identifying doctors personally rather than places (institutions) as sources of care, and people with lower rather than higher drug costs are higher self-medicators (Bush and Rabin, 1976). Smokers more often self-medicate than do non-smokers (Seltzer, Friedman and Sieglaub, 1974).

Self-medicators tend to be interested in health (read health articles, believe in medical examinations), ask pharmacists for advice and report themselves as having some illness or discomfort, but not as being in poor health. Tiredness, aches, digestive disorder, upper respiratory infections and depression are recent symptoms associated with being a self-medicator. They do not go to faith healers (Johnson *et al.*, 1976).

Among upper and middle income groups, being healthy but simultaneously experiencing aches and pains (headaches, muscle pain, etc.) is associated with higher OTC remedy use, and among rich and poor (not middle income groups) rate of use increases with the severity of acute illness. Generally those taking non-prescribed drugs are more likely to be using prescriptions as well; when looking only at those reporting themselves as ill, self-medication is associated with less prescription drug use. These same people have fewer doctor visits (Bush and Rabin, 1976).

When economic factors are controlled, that is when there is no cost to the consumer in visiting a doctor, this use of OTC substances presumably in lieu of a doctor visit is maintained for adults but not for children (Dunnell and Cartwright, 1972). Wadsworth *et al.* (1971)

also report that socio-economic class is rarely found to be a major factor in medical visits (in Western countries). Consistent with this, Smith (1976) reports that failure of patients (in Wisconsin) to purchase prescriptions ordered for them by doctors was not related either to the price of the medicine or the patients' income. These general observations may not hold true for the very poor. Smith (1976) reported that the institution of a Medicaid prescription drug payment plan in the southern United States significantly increased the number of prescriptions obtained in the community: the impact of Medicaid has been positive in increasing accessibility to medical care, at least for the very poor.

Blum and Associates (1972) in a study of normal drug use in a California urban population found that most persons commonly employed OTC and licit psychoactives, that there was a correlation between licit and illicit drug use rates, that present use correlated with lifetime experience (i.e. present with past experience), that greater licit drug use was associated with greater utilisation of medical care, more belief in the efficacy of medication, and in offering drugs to others (i.e. in the home or to friends). People in the greater drug use group were more often 'ill' (self-reported) as children and found advantage in taking the patient role. Greater drug experience is also correlated with psychological conflicts centred about orality as measured by reported eating problems, both as children and adults.

Age is one factor repeatedly associated with variations in medicine use. Dunnell and Cartwright (1972) found that the elderly and children under two had the most symptoms reported (children by their parents) and were the biggest consumers of both OTC and prescription medicines. Knoben and Wertheimer (1976) describe the pattern of drug consumption in the US as a function of ageing, dropping sharply after the first few years of life, and then gradually increasing until, in the elderly,[1] it approximates the rate of use for infants. The nature of drugs most commonly used changes drastically though. With prescriptions, for example, over 20 per cent of those for children under ten are for cough and cold remedies; anti-infective drugs constitute over 50 per cent of the 100 most frequently prescribed drugs for persons under 20. Oral contraceptives account for almost half of the drugs prescribed in the 20-39 age group, while 25 per cent of the top 100 drugs are cardiovascular agents in the population aged 65 and over.

Approximately 20 per cent of all prescriptions for people over 20 are for psychoactive drugs. When self-administered these drugs show marked differences in rates of use by age; this factor is interacting with a variety of other psychosocial factors (Blum *et al.*, 1972).

With regard to the issue of self-medication as a substitute for or supplement to medical care, the Johnson *et al.* and Bush and Rabin interpretations are contrary. The former argue that since OTC use occurs most among the healthy, self-limiting with minor discomforts, it is, assuming the efficacy of self-medication, rational. The latter investigators, although finding a similar phenomenon in one population group, find, as do Dunnell and Cartwright, a second group, the self-reported acutely ill who self-medicate without seeing a doctor. They argue that substitution is occurring even though most of the acute symptoms are self-limiting ones. Implicit is the possibility that some apparently self-limiting acute illnesses may require medical care.

Explicit in Bush and Rabin is the argument of risk; they describe findings by Hodes and Fonaroff to the effect that 19 per cent of ingestions reported to a poison centre were of non-prescribed medicines. They would also deny the rationality of self-medication on grounds of evidence for efficacy, citing the US National Academy of Sciences/National Research Council review of 400 OTC drugs, where it was found that only 42 per cent of the substances were effective or probably effective. US Food and Drug Administration panels reviewing antacids, sleep aids, and stimulants have been critical of all (except caffeine) as unsafe or inappropriate. Their further argument is economic, that much OTC use is wasteful of resources, a response of consumers to advertising.

Bush and Rabin do grant that substitution can be appropriate, that by providing relief to those with discomfort who, were they to visit a doctor, would strain the medical care system and increase the cost of that system to taxpayers or the paying patient.

In advanced technological societies, the issue of substitution of self-medication (as a presumed bad) versus the supplemental use of non-prescribed substances seems, on the evidence, of little consequence. Insofar as medical care is widely available, those who do not utilise it are likely to be influenced by forces additional to the simplicity and cheapness of home remedies and OTC compounds. Morris (1957) found that Englishmen most in need of care were often those who resisted both preventive medicine and illness care visits. In societies where medical care is not readily available, the issue of substitution of self-care for prescriptions is moot; people will do what they can to feel better — including utilising the remedies and rituals of folk medicine or hints of knowledge filtered down from scientific and technological spheres. The latter, when it comes to buying powerful medications as OTC substances in regions with insufficient regulation, will most probably be more dangerous than the panoply of folk practices.

As regards the reasons that citizens in technologically advanced societies do sometimes prefer to self-medicate when they should seek medical advice, the research to date is suggestive but insufficient. Surveys and questionnaires, the most employed methods, lead to only one level of knowledge. One can posit, on the basis of what has been shown, the existence within persons of at least two kinds of orientations and judgements affecting medication propensities. One factor seems to be perceived illness severity and health status. That is, of course, dependent on cultural and family definitions of health role interference (Zola, 1973) posed by the condition, what one has learned from doctors (see Balint, 1957, on their 'apostolic' function) on how to handle illness, perhaps anxiety thresholds linked to pain (an extensive literature shows that pain tolerance varies widely) and to felt psychological needs to suppress or seek assistance for distress. Zborowski (1952) has shown, for example, that whether or not and how people express themselves when in pain varies systematically from culture to culture. It is not unlikely that both doctor visiting and drug use are related to such cultural-psychological-physiological matters.

A second factor — really a basket for a variety of psychological variables — suggested by extant studies derives from the apparent correlation between health interests (or preoccupations), prescription, OTC and even illicit drug use, past pleasure in the childhood illness role, orality conflicts expressed in past eating problems (obesity, childhood finickiness, etc.) and beliefs in the 'power' of medicines, as opposed for example (see Johnson *et al.*, 1976) to faith healers. This pot-pourri of clearly psychodynamic variables suggests that more than advertising or a 'rational' knowledge of medicines costs or drug safety and efficacy will be found to influence people's self-medicating, as well as their other health practices. Indeed, a person can be quite 'rational' about evaluating drug effects and reach conclusions contrary to clinical or experimental investigators simply by virtue of experiencing the placebo effect, capable of occurring in 30 or 40 per cent of a population, and shown to be a function of setting, expectations and personality (Kornetsky, 1976). It does seem then that a fertile field for investigation will be that of psychological influences prompting medicines' use or rejection.

Information and Education

There is much emphasis on the provision of information to consumers/ patients as a means for influencing individual drug use conduct. Implicit is the model of the rational human; given facts on medicines, for example, indications, side effects, manner of use, contraindications, best buys, etc., it is assumed that people will act in their own self-interest by utilising that information. If an individual does not act wisely on the basis of information available then at least — so it is argued — the information provider has done his duty or, in countries with laws requiring 'informed consent' or 'full disclosure', the information provider has at least protected himself by obeying the law. Thus, one sees that information provision may have several different objectives (Wickware, 1977; Salisbury, 1977).

There is no agreement to the effect that information is a good thing or that consumers should be informed. Two paths of dissent are seen; one is offered by physicians who claim essentially that knowledge is a dangerous thing. It is feared that the informed patient will become frightened as he learns what harm medicine can do; fright can lead either to failure to take prescribed medicine or to time-consuming questions, overreporting of side-effects or upsetting emotional exchanges. One sees evidence of the information-is-dangerous view in the US patient package inserts (PPIs) legislation, recently debated and passed. Wickware (1977) reports a poll of physicians in which opponents outnumbered advocates two to one. Some physician comments are quoted below:

'The PPI would probably stimulate a lot of unnecessary questions . . . Drug use and hazard information are best given by the physician and pharmacist, who can make allowances for individual patient's needs and intelligence.'

'My telephone is already an "occupational hazard". I can see myself being obliged to give minicourses in medicine and pharmacology.'

'As a physician I'm an expert . . . We must not confuse patient education . . . with medical education which has no business being directed at patients.'

'In my experience, so-called informed patients are often the most difficult to treat.'

'Patients already know more than is good for them. I get tired of explaining to my patients.'

'Trust is the key word between physician and patient . . . my patients trust me to protect them.'

'This is my responsibility, not the patient's.'

Statements to the contrary have been made:

'The patient is now considered to be a member of the health care team' (Eric Martin, FDA).

'Patients (are) seeking, or demanding, or having thrust upon them an increasing role in clinical decision-making' (Dana Wickware).

Review of the opponents' remarks allows the inference that some physicians have self-images and concepts of the relationship with patients which restrict communication. One is reminded of earlier studies (Blum *et al.*, 1972) which identified some physicians more likely than their colleagues to arouse dissatisfaction in their patients, needing to feel superior to their patients, to command rather than discuss, and to require gratitude rather than shared decisions.

A complementary patient role was found in which patients wanted to be passive, not responsible, disinterested in information and looking up to the doctor as a father or god-like figure. These findings from the 1950s, mirrored in the 1977 remarks about PPIs, indicate that intra- and interpersonal psychological features will strongly influence what is communicated about medicines, when and how. As with much communication, the message may not be in the content of words. Relevant here is Davis' (1968) factorial study of 223 doctor-patient interactions which identifies ten patterns of interaction, some of which facilitate and some obstruct the flow of information both ways between doctor and patient. Seen in this context, 'information-providing' seems to be the function of a rather complex setting. Such a setting would necessitate taking into account doctors' and patients' characteristics as well as the peculiarities of their role-playing when working out a programme for improvement of patients' behaviour towards medicines.

A second source of resistance to informing consumers is to be inferred from the legislative process and the content of advertising.

Full disclosure about the limitations of medicines, either on prescription or OTC, is not readily drawn from many manufacturers. Instead the tendency is to broaden indications, minimise dangers and exaggerate efficacy. The reason is profit-making.

There is a muddy area conceptually in the literature on information. It has to do with the information in contrast to education. We have not found a clear statement as to intended difference in meaning; implicit, it appears, is a short-term or one-shot act of disclosure undertaken without regard to impact, that being information, and a long-term programme intended to produce broad changes in understanding and behaviour: education.

Intent, of course, is not fact and the assumption made by the health educator or consumer informant that he or she is producing wiser behaviour in another person must be tested by empirical research. Such research requires careful design, as Green (1977) has observed. At its best, such study will identify the variables associated with both varying effects and possibly different reasons for ineffectiveness in information and education programmes. As communication studies show in general, impact varies with the nature and the source of the material, means of communication, setting, relationship between communicator and subject, and the characteristics of the subject (prior exposure, interest, intelligence, personality, etc.). A wealth of studies show that response of persons to their environment, including intellectual information, is complexly determined indeed with un-conscious and subliminal processes operating as well as conscious ones.

With respect to the response to drug information, most work has been in the field of compliance, the study of factors influencing the degree to which a patient conforms to his doctors' prescription recommendation. There are in addition a few studies of consumer characteristics associated with health knowledge levels, and a few observations on response to new programmes, for example, clinical pharmacy or drug information centres. Lasagna and Joubert (1975) for example report that health knowledge and information levels about medicines vary inversely with age and directly with respect to social and educational levels. That finding is in keeping with a general principle derived from social research to the effect that as social class increases, so does formal education and, concomitantly, information about most public matters, participation and activity in community affairs, and sophistication in family and self-care.

In societies with few barriers to job and educational mobility, personal features such as motivation and intelligence will, in turn, affect class membership; so too will those variables which affect opportunity, for example, parental aspirations, residence, and adverse features such as discrimination, rigid tradition, political controls, or vocational and educational resource inadequacies. The point to be made here is that health knowledge, including information about medicines, is but one instance of that general sophistication which is predictable on the basis of economic, social, political and personal factors which affect the availability of, access to, interest in, and capacity to utilise knowledge sources.

As to the general state of medicines' sophistication, even within research and health orientated societies, little data is available. Knapp, Baird and Winter (1976) in a Food and Drug Administration study do report among American consumers healthy scepticism about both advertising and the safety and efficacy of OTC medicines. At the same time, paradoxically, large numbers are said to believe that preparations sold over the counter without prescriptions are harmless. Such inconsistencies are not atypical and suggest that people can adhere to several beliefs at once; the incompatibility judgement depending upon the information available to an observer. Lasagna (1969) for example, in the course of investigating the effect of extensive information about drugs and consumers' willingness to take them, reported that when all of the possible dangers and side effects of aspirin were made known to study participants, but the identity of the drug withheld, a high percentage declined to take the drug. When informed that the drug was aspirin, few people expressed reluctance to take it in spite of the side effect warnings. The dynamics of such contraindications can be understood through further study; one speculates that in the foregoing aspirin study, stereotypes of safety may overrule new information; similarly personal experience of low risks could well account for disregarding warnings. Again that is compatible with general research findings; when people's experiences have been good they are reluctant to accept warnings as to future dangers, especially if those would disrupt customary, satisfactory behaviour (Blum, 1956).

Of relevance here is the finding reported by Soueif (1967) that danger — in this instance punishment by incarceration — was effective as a deterrent against continuous cannabis consumption in only a very small percentage of long-term cannabis users (ranging between 6 per cent and 14 per cent). Similarly, Hammond (1963) reported that only 6.3 per cent of a large group of tobacco smokers were ready to give up smoking because of the propagated scientific information as to the association between smoking and lung cancer (Matarazzo and Saslow, 1960). Clearly, future risk does not weigh strongly in the balance against present pleasure with reference to ingrained ingestion habits. Overeating is a further illustration.

How much information should consumers have about prescription drugs they are taking? Lasagna and Joubert (1975) report that according to patients' perceptions, pharmacists and physicians are only partially and inadequately educating patients about drugs. In a study by Pratt *et al.* (1958) of physician-patient interaction, it was found that patients had less knowledge than they wanted about health matters and less knowledge than their doctors thought they should have. While patients had a realistic assessment of their state of knowledge, doctors generally underestimated the knowledge their patients did have. The more the physician underrated the knowledge of a patient, the less he explained about the patient's condition; and the less a patient knew, the fewer questions he asked. However, patients who received some explanation were more likely to increase their understanding and tended to ask more questions.

Although the physician was the generally preferred source of information, younger, more educated persons and those who were not in regular contact with a doctor placed greater importance on non-physician sources of information. Persons who did not regularly see a physician desired more information about drugs than those who saw a doctor regularly (Lasagna and Joubert, 1975).

Many countries now encourage or require informational patient package inserts to accompany prescription drugs dispensed to the consumer. In addition to supplying the consumer with information he did not previously have about drugs and his health, such devices may open lines of communication between medical practitioners and patients by providing a basis of consumer knowledge from which he can begin to ask questions of medical professionals.

Lasagna and Joubert (1975) found an inverse relationship between the volume of information and degree of the consumer's comprehension and, further, that complete information on all possible side effects can make some people excessively fearful. As a compromise, they suggest that a short summary of important drug information be included along with the longer more detailed version, for those who wish more information, and that benefits as well as risk information be included. They emphasise that the patient package insert should be written in simple, clear, layman's language to be accessible to a wide population and that more research is necessary to determine the optimum format and contents for the inserts.

With reference to reactions of US women to the mandatory insert which accompanies oral contraceptives, the consumer audience is receptive to and desirous of such information. A study of Fleckenstein (1976) of over 700 women users or previous users of oral contraceptives showed that 90 per cent of the women read the insert and 86 per cent considered it useful. Reported reading of the package insert was associated with a high score on a quiz about pill use and side effects; 70 per cent of the population, however, considered the insert inadequate by itself and desired more information from professionals. In addition, considerable anxiety was found over the possibility of serious side effects; 44 per cent of all women questioned, felt that the risks outweighed the benefits, including almost one-third of the current users, an unexplained inconsistency. The author notes that risk factors are emphasised far more than benefits, however, and concluded that there is a need for a more balanced, thorough presentation of information from educated health professionals.

Marsha Cohen, spokesperson for the US Consumers Union, reports (1976) that the CU advocates that the following information be available on the patient package insert: care of medicine, warnings (such as 'habit-forming'), possible side effects, significant contraindications, generic and brand name of drug, strength, expiry date, and explicit directions for use. Patient medication cards, developed by a few hospitals, generally carry this information in abbreviated form, and include instructions on which side effects are serious and indicate that the medicine should be discontinued and a physician consulted.

Objective Sources

It is likely that most of the information which consumers receive is, in societies with profit-oriented pharmaceutical industries, biased in favour of products. Certainly the budgets for advertising exceed funds available for public health or educational programmes, and the amount of time for which the consumer is exposed to biased materials will be greater than his exposure to objective drug information from pharmacists, doctors or health educators. There are, unfortunately, no studies which compare the impact of biased as opposed to objective sources.

A few studies do bear on objective information programmes. A major effort in England and the US has been to train clinical pharmacists as information givers, or to provide, experimentally, pharmacy information centres available for telephone or write-in questions. McKenney (1973) and others report on the potential gains from such activities, and studies of compliance (see later section) show their impact. One must not assume, however, that 'objective' sources are either objective or wise. Jackson and Smith (1974) discovered that when a prescription for coumarin was obtained and aspirin was requested by the same client, half of the pharmacists studied failed to alert the buyer to the potentially deadly interaction between the two.

School efforts and community campaigns offer tests of the impact of health education. Woodcock (in Blum, Blum and Garfield, 1976), reviewing the health education evaluation findings, is not optimistic about that impact. There are two studies, however, which demonstrated change. In one, Farquhar and Maccoby (1975) undertook three different education approaches in three relatively similar Californian towns, the goal being to alter life-styles with higher risks of cardiac disease (overweight, smoking, cholesterol high diets, no exercise, etc.). They were able, through advertising and group involvement, significantly to alter citizen behaviour in the direction of healthier living. In another study on the educational impact of classroom presentation on children's non-medical drug use, Blum, Blum and Garfield (1976) showed that education, over a two-year period, did change childrens' drug use in the direction of reduced use of un-sanctioned substances such as heroin, LSD or barbiturates. It was also found, however, that such education speeded up experimentation with more socially acceptable compounds such as alcohol, tobacco, and cannabis. Neither of these studies are of medicines' use per se; they do offer hope of the possibility of successful consumer education by school and community health programmes.

Consumer Advertising

The effects of OTC advertising have been widely and heatedly debated, particularly advertising on television, since TV is rated (by most Americans) as the most believable mass medium (Roper 1973). One out of every eight commercial spots on television is for some OTC remedy, and four out of the top five television advertisers are drug companies (National Council of Churches Report on Hearings on Drug Advertising, 1973).

In a study by Peterson and others (1976) where commercials were monitored, it was found that no contraindications for use or side effects are mentioned in the advertising. Raters judged 80 per cent of the advertisements as encouraging pill-taking and suggesting casual use of drugs. In a study conducted with teenage boys in the US over a period of three years, National Association of Broadcasters' researchers found a weak positive relationship between TV exposure and the boys' reported use of OTC medicines, and a stronger correlation in cases where there were more OTC drugs in the home (Milanski *et al.*, 1975).

Self-policing of commercials by the industry has been only marginally successful. Peterson *et al.* (1976) compared drug commercials before and after National Association of Broadcasters guidelines went into effect, and found that there was no significant decrease in violation of the guidelines that 'drugs be presented for occasional use only' and that spots should 'not suggest casual use of drugs'. Although the degree to which advertising influences drug misuse or overuse has not yet been scientifically established, it can reasonably be asserted that the intense promotion of OTC drugs contributes to public misconceptions about the utility and need for drugs, and reinforces values, and attitudes which encourage drug use. Peterson *et al.* (1976), Roper (1973), National Council of Churches (1973) and Farquhar and Maccoby (1975) showed that mass media campaigns have affected behaviour as well as attitudes. A possibly more significant, though subtle, contribution of advertising is its characterisation of everyday stress and discomfort as a medical problem which is amenable to treatment and that seeking treatment or relief in drugs is desirable and even unselfish (Lennard and Epstein *et al.*, 1971).

In a petition to the FDA, Marsha Cohen, consultant to the Consumers Union of the US, Inc., observed that since advertising of OTCs does not disclose risks, warnings and contraindications, the package insert is often ignored because of the 'safety image' created by the media. In addition, this information is not available to the consumer until after purchase, so the consumer, having spent his money anyway, may decide to take the chance and use the medicine in spite of the warnings. The CU advocates that advertising include all relevant warnings and contraindications in serial, if necessary – that is with one or two information items included in each commercial spot – so that full exposure is achieved within a given period of time; it also advocates that advertisements should not make claims which the FDA will not allow on labels and package inserts.

Control of OTC drugs and advertising has been argued. Currently in the US, efforts are being made to co-ordinate jurisdiction and requirements for labelling, which has been the FDA's responsibility, and contents of promotion and advertising, which has traditionally been the responsibility of the Federal Trade Commission.

In Norway, all commercial drug information is controlled before a drug firm is allowed to send it out. No advertising of drugs is permitted on television or in public places. The effectiveness of these measures has, however, not been evaluated.

The European Public Health Committee has made several recommendations to decrease the abuse of OTC medicines, including wide distribution of information and guidelines on how OTCs should be used, and education by physicians and pharmacists directed at consumers. Their proposed government interventions include assurance that OTC drugs on the market are safe and efficacious, that they include stable and clear-cut indications for use, and that advertising be limited to clear factual claims.

Information vs. Regulation

The number of many OTC drugs in the home is modestly correlated with an increased responsiveness of adolescents to commercial TV advertising. Similarly, use by parents of psychoactive drugs — either on prescription or recreationally (as with cocktails) — has been shown to be correlated with the readiness of their children to take such substances illicitly. One suspects the existence of a facilitating milieu characterised by drug availability, drug acceptance, and the teaching — by mass media and the family — of medicine use.

Given the facilitation of drug use through learning from the parental model, it is reasonable to ask if safety with respect to drugs can also be learned. Certainly the studies on recreational drugs, alcohol in particular, suggest that children growing up in cultural environments where safe drinking habits are taught by parents will indeed be immunised against later alcoholism.

Strong evidence can be derived that safety can better be achieved via regulation than via information. More carefully stated when prior information simply advising safety has not been effective, one can say there is inferential evidence, at least in one population sector, to the effect that the risk of harm can be dramatically reduced by physical security measures. The illustration is drawn from childhood poisoning from drugs in the home.

Dunnell and Cartwright (1972) found that in over two-thirds of the homes surveyed in England, medicines were not locked up. In the US, children in school and parents via mass media and labels, have long been advised to keep medicines secure from young children;

nevertheless, poisoning deaths continued. Then in the US the use of safety packaging was introduced in 1970. It became mandatory for manufacturers and pharmacists, to dispense aspirin and all prescription medicines in containers difficult for a small child (and for many adults!) to open. As McIntire, Angle and Grush (1976) report, there was a dramatic effect on accidental poisonings. Protection via regulation succeeded where education and information warnings failed. The exception has been, according to McIntire *et al.*, the older child with a history of prior poisoning.

In small population tests of one child-resistant package closure, the incidence of poisoning by prescription drugs was diminished over 75 per cent (Breault, 1974; Scherz, 1974). In the US the Poison Prevention Act of 1970 made child-proof packaging mandatory for aspirin and all prescription medicines. Accidental poisoning deaths due to aspirin dropped 50 per cent in the year following implementation and the most recent statistics indicate a downward tend in poisoning due to prescription drugs (Garrettson, 1977). The public has shown a high level of acceptance of safety packaging (McIntire, 1977).

The poisoning data do not show that informing people about drug hazards does not work, after all most children do not poison themselves and presumably at least some parents (up to one-third, if one uses the Dunnell and Cartwright study as a baseline) may have learned medicine safety. This natural experiment does show that physical prevention mandated by law can have a dramatic impact on consumer safety when ordinary information efforts have failed. The inherent limits of mandatory measures is most readily seen in the drug abuse arena or in the case of cancer remedies such as Laetrile where, in the US, even criminal penalties have not prevented cancer patients from illegally importing and using this substance, which has been termed totally ineffective by the FDA; obviously, when medicines have high symbolic value or are pleasure-producing, regulation and information may both be inadequate means for influencing consumer behaviour.

Patient Compliance with Medicine Regimen

People taking prescription medicines often do not follow their physicians' instructions for consumption of the drugs. This phenomenon is of concern to many health care providers and observers. The term 'compliance' has most often been used to describe patients' consumption of medicines as directed. This term has the disadvantage

Table 6.1: Factors which have been Found to Affect Conformity to Physicians' Prescriptions

Factor Class	Factor	Association with Conformity
socio-demographic	age over 65	negative
	extreme youth	negative
disease	psychiatric diagnosis	negative
medication regimen	frequency of doses	negative
	complexity of schedule	negative
	number of drugs	negative
	degree of behavioural change required	negative
	duration of therapy	variable (*may* affect)
	drug class or type of drug	negative (*may* affect)
	side effect	
patient-therapist interaction	degree of supervision	positive
	patient dissatisfaction	negative
	good communication	positive (*may* affect)
patient characteristics	'appropriate' health beliefs	positive
	personality disorder	negative
	extremely high or low anxiety levels	negative
	perception of ill health/efficacy of medicine	positive
	health knowledge	negative
	drug knowledge	negative
other	social isolation	negative
	family stability	positive
	family supportiveness/positive attitude towards therapy	positive

of being value-laden, implying that a submissive, obedient role is appropriate for the patient. In discussing PPIs, the dispute about the patient role *vis à vis* the physician has been mentioned. The 'compliance' literature demonstrates that emotions and communications locked to role behaviour do strongly influence patients' use of medicine.

The quality of that literature is disappointing because of badly desgined studies, inadequate controls, poor execution and the inherent complexity of the phenomenon. Most studies fall below acceptable levels in these areas, and many are not reported in sufficient detail to determine their quality. In the balance, however, some conclusions can be reached. Keep in mind that the more accurate the measure of compliance, and the more strict the interpretation of 'compliance' the higher is the rate of discrepancy observed between what patients do and what a doctor's prescription calls for in manner (frequency, dose, duration, etc.) of medicine use (Sackett and Haynes, 1976).

Generally more than 50 per cent of the study population do not consume medicines as directed by their physicians; in some the rate exceeded 80 per cent. One well-designed study of outpatients in a teaching hospital disclosed that only 22 per cent of the prescriptions were being consumed as directed and over 30 per cent were being 'mis-utilised in a manner that posed a serious threat to the patient's health' (Boyd *et al.*, 1974).

Patients' variation from expected drug regimens is attributable to many factors, including some which may not be explicit in the physician's instructions, for example, using old medicine for a new order or self-medicating with old medicines. Dunnell and Cartwright (1972) report that over 25 per cent of the adults interviewed took leftover medicines as late as a year after it had been prescribed.

Studies have yielded a number of factors which have been found to affect conformity to physicians' prescriptions (see Table 6.1).

Determinants of Compliance

Non-compliance can be attributed to patients' misunderstanding of prescription directions (Hermann, 1973; Mazzullo *et al.*, 1974). Mazzullo, Lasagna and Griner (1974) found that not once in their study was a prescription label interpreted uniformly by all patients. Many labels did contain ambiguous directions, yet those with directions which were considered explicit were frequently misinterpreted. Even when patients were given written instructions to take home with them, instructions which named the medicine and told of its use, less than two-thirds knew the name of the medicine being taken, and only three-quarters accurately reported the medicine's use. The average patient in this study (Hladik and White, 1976) did not recall instructions as to when to take the medicine or under what circumstances to change dosage.

In addition to explicitness versus ambiguity, comprehensibility versus incomprehensibility of directions must be considered. Empirical testing of comprehensibility of instructions by representatives of the target recipients should be the rule. Ley *et al.* (1972) applied Flesch's formula for estimating the percentage of population who would be capable of understanding a piece of written material in X-ray leaflets issued by a hospital which received most of its clients from a lower working-class district. The leaflets were found to be very difficult to understand. Similar findings were reported by Lovius *et al.* (1973) with regard to leaflets issued by a dental hospital.

There is some evidence to the effect that ensuring comprehensibility of written directions makes the picture more optimistic. Ley (1977) studied the effects of increased comprehension on accuracy of medicine-taking in psychiatric patients. It was claimed that easily and moderately comprehensible instructions were found to be correlated with behavioural compliance with the doctor's instructions. On the other hand, material difficult to comprehend was found ineffective in reducing errors in medicine-taking behaviour.

Hassar (1976) followed up on patients who had been given an information sheet prior to securing their informed consent (signed) as participants in a trial of an anti-inflammatory drug. Hassar found that two-thirds of the patients did not remember that they had been told (and given reading material about) the risk of gastrointestinal ulceration. Hassar's findings, like those of Robinson and Merav (1976), pertaining to informed consent in surgery, show not only that patients may not recall the essentials of risk information, but also deduce incorrect conclusions and remain otherwise misinformed, this in spite of their signatures on the consent form. One must conclude that even when physician's instructions are reinforced by written take-home instructions and consent forms, there is no assurance that the patient will hear, read, or remember as important what the physician or researcher would think important.

Ley (1977) reviewed a number of studies pertinent to the problem of recall of instructions. Different categories of patients whose recall of advice given by their doctors, at various intervals ranging between a few minutes and a few weeks, after receiving the advice were found to forget quite a sizeable proportion of the instructions received, ranging between 37.2 per cent and 54 per cent. Interesting, also is the finding reported by Ley and Spelman (1967), later confirmed by Ley *et al.* (1976), that patients show a tendency to forget advice and instructions more frequently than other sorts of medical information given by their doctors. By manipulating relevant variables (i.e. importance of instructions as felt by patients, and the serial position of such instructions in the total material presented by the doctor), however, Ley could improve the percentage of instructions recalled by the patients (op. cit.).

Are there patient traits which predict compliance? Two studies report that there are. Eva Blum (1958) compared personality traits of behaviourally-identified co-operative and non-co-operative patients and developed a personality test which proved accurate in determining in advance which patients would be unco-operative with their doctors. Bakker and Dightman (1964) report that among women taking oral contraceptives, those who failed regularly were found to be more irresponsible, immature and impulsive than their conformant counterparts, factors similar to those observed by Blum.

Are there doctor-patient patterns of interaction which predict patients' compliance? Davis' study (1968) suggests there are. In a methodologically sophisticated work, Davis analysed patterns of doctor-patient interactions as measured by Bales' technique of interaction process analysis. Principal component analysis followed by rotation to oblique simple structure yielded 10 meaningful factors, which were interpreted as representing different patterns of doctor-patient interaction. Factor scores were computed for each doctor-patient pair to allow estimating correlation with weighted measures of patient compliance or conformance. Four of the factors had negative relationships with compliant behaviour. One factor had a positive correlation with patients' compliance. It should be noted that the correlations were not high. Nevertheless, the importance of this work lies in the fact that it draws attention to complex interpersonal determinants of patients' compliance.

Strong factors associated with compliance are patient health beliefs, such as the perception of severity of ill health, and satisfaction with doctor-patient interaction. Although the medical evaluation of the severity of a disease or condition does not correlate with prescription performance (Charney *et al.*, 1967; Hulka *et al.*, 1976; Johansen *et al.*, 1966; Bonner *et al.*, 1969; Davis, 1968), the patient's perception of the severity of resusceptibility to the disease (in paediatric cases, the

Figure 6.1: Hypothesised Model for Predicting and Explaining Compliance Behaviour

| Readiness to Undertake Recommended Compliance Behaviour | Modifying and Enabling Factors | Compliant Behaviours |

Motivations:
Concern about (salience of) health matters in general
Willingness to seek and accept medical direction
Intention to comply
Positive health activities

Value of Illness Threat Reduction:
Subjective estimates of:
Susceptibility or resusceptibility (including belief in diagnosis)
Vulnerability to illness in general
Extent of possible bodily harm*
Extent of possible interference with social roles*
Presence of (or past experience with) symptoms

Probability that Compliant Behaviour will Reduce the Threat:
Subjective estimates of:
The proposed regimen's safety
The proposed regimen's efficacy to prevent, delay or cure (incl. 'faith in doctors and medical care' and 'chance of recovery'

Demographic (very young or old)
Structural (cost, duration, complexity, side effects, accessibility of regimen, need for new patterns of behaviour)
Attitudes (satisfaction with visit, physician, other staff, clinic procedures and facilities)
Interaction (length, depth, continuity, mutuality of expectation, quality and type of doctor/patient relationship; physician agreement with patient; feedback to patient)
Enabling (prior experience with action, illness or regimen; source of advice and referral (incl. social pressure))

Likelihood of:
Compliance with preventive health recommendations and and prescribed regimens: *e.g.* screening, immunisations, prophylactic exams, drugs, diet, exercise, personal and work habits, follow-up tests, referrals and follow-up appointments, entering or continuing a treatment programme

*At motivating, but not inhibiting, levels.

mother's perceptions) correlate closely with conforming behaviour in a variety of populations studied. In most cases, belief that the medicine would be effective in curing or preventing recurrence of the disease was also associated with compliance.

Becker and Maiman (1975) have developed a belief model to describe compliance behaviour which is shown in Figure 6.1. (See also *Drug Therapy*, 1976.) Unco-operative patients, sampled from a range of medical specialties, proved to be less interpersonally effective, more maladjusted, more unrealistic in their expectations of medical care. There was evidence that unco-operativeness was a general rather than specific response to medical care (Eva Blum, 1958).

Satisfaction with doctor-patient interaction has been investigated in several studies. Three of these have produced evidence that the mother's satisfaction with a doctor in the paediatric clinic setting is an important factor in her conformance to physician recommendations. (Francis *et al.*, 1969; Becker *et al.*, 1971; Korsch and Negrete, 1972.) Korsch and Negrete (1972) found that the mother's satisfaction was not correlated with her educational level, the length of the session with the doctor, or the quality of the doctor's interaction with her child. The factors which correlated with both her satisfaction and a high level of compliance were the doctor's attention to her concerns, positive emotions towards her, and a reassuring attitude. Francis *et al.* (1969) report that most dissatisfied mothers were those who expected but did not receive an explanation of the causation and nature of their child's illness. This group was found to be significantly less compliant.

Becker and Green (1972) review work on the role of the family in influencing members' sick role behaviour and compliance with medical regimen, though not directly attending to adherence to medication intructions. For instance, Heinzelman and Bagley (1970) found that a man's pattern of adherence to a physical fitness plan designed to prevent a heart attack was directly related to his wife's attitude towards the programme. Since compliance with medication regimens has been found to correlate positively with observance of other medical recommendations, these findings of the important role of the support of the family members may well apply to pharmacotherapeutic regimes (Haynes, 1976 a and b).

Stokes and Dudley (1972) report that sex roles within marriage affected the couple's efficiency in the use of birth control methods. Couples who experienced maximum male-female role differentiation and little shared decision-making were less effective in contraceptive use, regardless of the method chosen. Undesired pregnancy rates were higher for couples with segregated conjugal roles even though they were at least as likely to use birth control pills or IUDs as their counterparts whose roles were less rigidly defined. The implication is that shared decision-making reduces conflict and facilitates effective behaviour. This also applies to the concept of 'informed consent' between physician and patient.

More fundamental than tailoring instructions to life style is the care given to instructing. Butt (1977) reviewing studies such as Nickerson (1972) in which 63 per cent of hospital released patients claimed they were given no self-care advice at all, emphasises that some communication must occur and that any methods to improve it are worth testing. Noting findings to the effect that recall is less than 50 per cent when instructions are given, that information retained does not increase the greater the amount provided by the physician, and that initial information is better retained than supplemental material, Butt provided patients with a cassette of the final meeting with the physician. Over 90 per cent of his sample said that they were helped by this device; the average replayed the interview three times. Using and being pleased does not, of course, demonstrate retention of facts or proper self-care. Hladik and White (1976), using a take-home card found that all of their follow-up cardiovascular patients said they read the materials and found them helpful; however, recall thereafter showed that most could not answer several questions about when and how to take their medicine.

Ley and his colleagues, who have done a number of studies in this area (see summary in Ley, P. *et al.*, 1976), conclude that patient dissatisfaction and failure to follow advice are related to failures to understand and remember. Seeking to remedy this, Ley *et al.* conducted a study in which physicians agreed to try to improve their communication, using a variety of methods. The results indicated that patients enjoying the elaborated communications did recall more, although instructions and advice were less well remembered than other conversation topics. Patients with a high comprehension of what had been said were higher in satisfaction and reported compliance. Paradoxically, however, comprehension improvement as such was not observed as a function of new communication styles (as we understand the data presented) even though item recall did improve and, thus, the experimental effort, while improving recall, did not improve comprehension, satisfaction or compliance. Only those blessed with an initially high comprehension had high satisfaction/compliance.

Improving Compliance

Several strategies have been tested for their capacity to improve compliance. Tailoring the medical regimen to the patient's life style, by linking dosage times to specific events in the patient's day, changing the form of a medicine from a liquid to a tablet for convenience, or where possible, substituting long-acting forms or combination drugs, have shown some promise. Fink (1976) claims significant improvement in clinical effectiveness of therapy for a study group whose regimens were so tailored; he emphasises however, the mutuality of the pharmacotherapist-patient relationship and the individuality of tailoring which presently make experimental replication and guidelines for implementation difficult. For example, in Fink's work it is difficult to tell how much improvement may be due to the tailored regimen, or to the individual attention and concern directed toward the now individualised patient care.

The Clinical Pharmacist

One of the proposed strategies for improving compliance as well as consumer safety has been the use of a clinical pharmacist who counsels the patient on how, and often why, he should consume his medicine. The pharmacist can do a check for physicians' prescription error or oversight. Counselling can range from a five-minute informational session, sometimes including written directions, to one or more lengthy conferences with the patient regarding problems with medications, new symptoms, diet, medicine (drug-drug) interactions and other health complaints. Success with use of clinical pharmacy services has been varied. An ongoing pharmacist monitoring programme for previously non-compliant hypertensive patients which included not only lengthy consultation and education but also blood pressure and weight checks, was successful in improving compliance for the duration of the study. When the programme was discontinued, non-compliance rates rose to their former levels. A 'no attention' placebo was used for the control group of patients in the study (McKenney *et al.*, 1973).

Several studies have indicated that one or two clinical pharmacy consultations have a significant effect on compliance but most do not include long-term follow-up (Madden, 1973; Cole and Emmanuel, 1971). Some simple instructions and reminder devices have proven significantly effective in improving compliance rates for short-term therapy (Mattar *et al.*, 1975; Sharpe and Mikeal, 1974; Clinite and Kabat, 1976; Lima *et al.*, 1976). In sum, it appears that informational efforts will not assure compliance improvement. On the other hand, clear and comprehensible directions for consumption in the context of doctor behaviour which increases patient satisfaction with the relationship, are prerequisities to improving the use of prescribed medicines by the consumer.

Physicians and the Prescribing of Drugs

Examining drug prescription patterns brings attention to what is termed 'drug misuse'. A major problem in developed countries in the West is that of 'overprescribing' of drugs, antibiotics and psychoactives (tranquillisers, sedatives and stimulants) in particular. Drugs are often prescribed in the absence of appropriate medical indications or for prolonged periods of time to relieve symptoms without an adequate diagnosis.

Antibiotics are the most improperly used drugs, as a class (*NY Times,* 1976). For example, an estimated 22 per cent of antibiotics used in hospitals are prescribed unnecessarily. In one study, no infection was present nor deemed likely to occur in 50 per cent of patients on antibiotic courses in a hospital; most of those were taking them as prophylactics, and a few antibiotics were prescribed on the basis of symptoms, though no infection was actually found. Lilja (1976) reports that when a sample of physicians were asked what they would prescribe for a theoretical case of pneumonia, 65 per cent chose a medically unsuitable drug. Moser (1964) reported that over half the antibiotics given to patients are not medically indicated, and that in a review of fatalities due to penicillin, use of that drug was not medically indicated in over half the cases. Stolley *et al.* (1972) found that 95 per cent of the physicians in their sample gave prescriptions to patients with a common cold, and 60 per cent of those prescriptions were for antibiotics, which are not effective in curing colds.

Part of this overuse may be due to physicians' lack of knowledge. In a test on antibiotic drugs by the Network for Continuing Medical Education, over half of the 4,000 doctors tested got fewer than 68 per cent of the examination questions correct. Schulz and Perrier (1976) found that 60 per cent of the interns they examined lacked the necessary pharmacological knowledge.

Physicians may not be unaware of their limitations and, indeed, may be anxious about prescribing. Julian and Herxheimer (1977), employing a training seminar method, attribute such anxieties to physicians' awareness of their lack of diagnostic skills, uncertainty about treatment, inexperience with the drug, and doubts about the ability to supervise or predict the patient's actual use of the medicine.

These physician inadequacies are not limited to pharmacotherapeutics alone, rather they illustrate one facet of human variability which, in the professional context, becomes a problem in the quality of care. Brook, Williams and Avery (1976), in a review of the physician quality literature, conclude that there are serious deficiencies in the US in medical care quality, including pharmacotherapeutics. Whilst quality differences are predictable on the basis of physician characteristics (younger, better trained MDs provide better care) the major problems seem to be in physician habits and health care locations and institutions as such. Efforts to improve care by providing knowledge to physicians have proved insufficient. The authors propose, in this article which should be read in its entirety, research on the measurement and rendering of quality care including better outcome measures and new disease taxonomies related to prognosis.

Insofar as their perspective is applicable outside the US, as it probably is, and applies to pharmacotherapeutics as much as to other areas of practice, the burden of improvement will depend on basic and applied research, and not on expanding present models based on inadequate assumptions as to how care is improved.

The misuse of medicines as such is not benign, nor merely wasteful in terms of money. The risk of superinfection from use of broad-spectrum antibiotics increases with the frequency of their use, as does the incidence of serious adverse drug reactions from almost any potent chemical entity. An investigation by McKenney and Harrison (1976) found that of 216 patients admitted to a general ward in a US teaching hospital, adverse drug reaction (ADR) was the cause of hospital admission of almost 8 per cent and, in 11 per cent an ADR was associated with the admission. ADRs were found to be the leading cause of drug-related hospital admission, ahead of non-compliance, inadequate therapy and drug overdose. An HEW report (Brodie, 1970) estimated that 1.5 million annual hospital admissions in the US are the result of adverse drug reactions. It is also estimated that 25 per cent of drugs prescribed in the US provide no patient benefit. (The 1974 NRC-NSF review of compounds on the market found that many were ineffective.)

Prescribing rates as to number of drugs prescribed per patient vary by nation. Among matched Scottish and American patients in university hospitals, Lawson (1976) found that drug therapy in America cost patients more in terms of financial outlay and adverse drug effects. American physicians tended to use more than one drug per specific indication or symptom, unlike their Scottish counterparts. Where American patients received an average of 9.1 drugs per hospital admission, Canadians average 7.1; Israelis 6.3; New Zealanders 5.8 and Scots 4.6.

Whether examined within or among nations, the competence and prescribing patterns of physicians are, no doubt, affected by many factors. These are distal determinants of the consumer's medical care and medicine use. At the least one expects drug availability, the adequacy of physician education, the integrity of pharmaceutical information given to the physician and the norms in the medical community to account for some of the differences between nations. Economic and regulatory factors are addressed elsewhere in this book.

By way of illustrative reference here, the findings of Wardell (1973) are noted; due to differing regulations on new drug development and marketing in the US and Britain, there is often a lag of up to several years between the introduction of drugs in Britain and their subsequent clearance for marketing in the United States. This has resulted in radically different clinical treatment patterns for patients with cardiac arrhythmia, for example, in the two countries. In some cases the lag has been detrimental to patients in the US. Delay also protects patients from prematurely marketed drugs.

In underdeveloped countries, a different set of problems emerge. Often, desperately needed medications are not available to consumers or practitioners. On the other hand, potent drugs may be marketed; few requirements exist on what information must accompany the drugs or advertisements. Indications for use, contraindication and side-effect warnings from the manufacturer are often incomplete and misleading where there is poor enforcement of, or lack of, adequate legislation over advertising and labelling. Moreover, powerful drugs are often 'prescribed' by untrained pharmacists and their assistants and are sold, in effect, over the counter. This situation is complicated by the lack of available trained medical personnel.

The classical case is misuse of chloramphenicol, a powerful, broad-spectrum antibiotic which was initially produced and marketed for a wide variety of indications. It was soon discovered that in 0.004 per cent of persons it caused a fatal and irreversible aplastic anaemia, and, in the US and Europe, its use was accordingly recommended only for specific diseases which were life-threatening and where other drugs were ineffectual, notably, typhoid fever and a specific form of meningitis.

Dunne, Herxheimer and others (1973) reviewed manufacturers' leaflets for 55 packs of the drug available in 29 countries and found wide disparities in information, including lists of unwarranted indications for use, and inadequate or non-existent warnings of the drug's dangers.[2] In the *Drugging of the Americas*, Silverman (1976) notes that chloramphenicol, like other drugs, is promoted to doctors by detail men not medically trained, as well as to untrained pharmacists who dispense the drug according to the detail men's directions. Evidence of chloramphenicol misuse for an upper respiratory infection in Latin American is manifested in fatal drug-induced aplastic anaemia. Chloramphenicol is of no use and dangerous in the treatment of upper respiratory infections.

It seems reasonable to suggest that the exposure of the physician to drug advertising plays a role in consumer safety, via prescriptions. Quite likely in settings where many professionals receive inadequate information, group norms build up and sanction what elsewhere may be considered malpractice. Such norms, once established, become 'traditions' and create barriers to improvement. Because of these social psychological factors, it is helpful to analyse physician behaviour in terms of group or organisational processes, as these affect prescribing.

Blum (1958) for example, found remarkable differences in the quality of medical care, and related subsequent patient dissatisfaction, depending on the organisation of hospitals: how physicians there selected and supervised themselves; how the institution ran; what emphasis there was on quality care; etc. Information flow, as defined by readiness to use particularly qualified consultants and feedback to physicians from audit committees was an important quality variable.

Coleman, Katz and Menzel (1966) describe two networks representing colleague interaction among physicians. Physicians at the hubs of the network of professional consultation, who were consulted more often by their colleagues, were innovators. Better informed and more active, they began prescribing new drugs earlier than those who were rarely consulted. A similar network for social interaction was also developed and found to have significant effects on prescribing. But while the professional network showed influences on prescribing immediately after the new drug was introduced, the social or friendship network appeared to reach its peak of influence in later months. Physicians who were professionally and socially integrated with their colleagues and within the formal structure of the health care system, and who had closer hospital or clinic affiliation were more influenced by interpersonal factors than were their isolated colleagues. Such studies show the influence of social network characteristics on physician information and subsequent patient care.

Other studies, for example, Blum's on malpractice (1957) show how personality features are also involved; indeed, personality factors influence the nature of physician's collegial relationships and thus their roles and placement in such professional and friendship networks.

Physicians' Prescribing Habits

Studies in this field, as in the area of compliance, are often inadequate, and limited in scope, as Hemminki (1976) points out. Official sales figures for drugs are not available in many countries, physicians are not often willing to talk about their prescribing habits and the drug industry 'is often unwilling to let outsiders study its activities and is unco-operative in giving information'. In spite of serious difficulties, some general features have emerged consistently in the prescribing literature and can shed some light on physicians' prescribing practices.

Joyce *et al.* (1968) and others (Becker *et al.*, 1971) found that higher educational qualifications were associated with lower prescribing of all kinds. Garner (1971) reported that specialists tend to prescribe more appropriately and conservatively, to search for specific cause of disease rather than to treat symptoms, and prescribed more single-entity, specific antibiotics than general practitioners who tended to use non-specific broad-spectrum ones.

Becker *et al.* (1971) investigated quality of prescribing, using frequency of prescriptions for chloramphenicol for a sample of 34 physicians. Because the medically legitimate uses for this drug are highly restricted, a lower prescribing rate is used as an index for appropriate prescribing. They found that physicians who prescribed chloramphenicol less frequently were more often in group practice, were younger, busier physicians with larger ancillary staffs, who had more postgraduate education and were more concerned with psycho-social aspects of medicine, were more willing to consult with and refer patients to other physicians and were more wary of pharmaceutical firms and detail men.

Conversely, those characteristics associated with high chloramphenicol use were a physician's solo practice, increased average age, isolation from colleagues, and reluctance to consult with or refer to other physicians. These physicians tended to be more willing to accept detail men and pharmaceutical firms as sources of information. Some of these same features are ones identified by Katz as linked to responsiveness to new findings in pharmacotherapeutics, and by Blum as linked to patient satisfaction and the risk of malpractice suits.

Freidson (1961) reported, in a study of prepaid medical group practice, that physicians in a group practice tend to keep in closer contact with their colleagues; and that institutional structure also provides an informal peer review of prescribing practice. The prepaid plan seems to also have the effect of allowing the physician to resist patients' unreasonable demands for drugs; since the physician is salaried and does not depend on the patient's continued patronage for his job, these factors need not interfere with his sound medical judgements.

Coleman *et al.* (1966) also found that informal discussion with colleagues played a role in the decision by a physician to prescribe a new drug. Friendship links were found to be more important in cities of 30,000 to 40,000 people than in a city of 110,000, though advisorship and partnership relationships remained unchanged in their influence. As in the Katz study, physicians who were socially isolated were slower to begin prescribing a new drug than those who were integrated into a social professional network.

Menzel and Katz found that physicians tended to consult colleagues more often in cases of chronic diseases, where there are many possible treatments and the outcome is more ambiguous than in cases of acute disease. Thus, one confirms that the social and professional relationships of physicians to their colleagues play a vital role in learning to prescribe.

A clarification of the importance of various sources of new drug information, including advertising, is made by Coleman *et al.* (1966) and analysed into stages of adoption of innovation by Miller. Miller's analysis may help clarify the role of detail men as influences on prescribing. The first stage in the descriptive model is 'awareness', where a physician is first alerted to a new medicine's availability. In about 75 per cent of the cases studied by Coleman, detail men and trade journals published by pharmaceutical manufacturers were found to be the primary sources of information at this point. In the second 'interest' stage, the physician's use of direct mail advertising and detail men declines and is replaced by consultation with colleagues, and by professional journals and journal advertising. In the third 'evaluation' stage, the use of these latter sources increases. Coleman's findings are generally supported by Ferber and Wales' diary reports from physicians in a different part of the country. The 'trial' stage is where the physician tries the drug on a limited number of patients to determine its value. The 'adoption' stage occurs when he begins prescribing the drug routinely to a whole class of patients. At these later stages, there is some evidence that, once again, printed material such as advertising becomes more important (Miller, 1973-4).

In time, Freidson has noted, a clinician is prone to give more weight to his own clinical experience rather than rely on 'book knowledge' or abstract principles. This observation is supported by the response of physician readers to a drug information survey. When asked what they would do if the bulletin printed a clearly adverse report on safety or efficacy of a new drug, most physicians responded that if the report concerned safety, they would discontinue use of the drug. If, however, the report concerned efficacy, they would trust their own clinical impressions (see also Ruskin, 1974).

This point of view may appear reasonable and fairly benign; however, we have previously discussed common patterns of the physician-patient relationship which may distort a physician's clinical impressions as well as deny the dangers associated with any potent drugs.

An extreme case of the negative aspect of physicians' trust in their own clinical impressions over controlled clinical trials is embodied in the case of DES (di-ethyl stilboestrol). From 1946 to 1970, a form of synthetic oestrogen was administered to pregnant women who were considered high risks for miscarriage. DES was claimed to prevent spontaneous abortion, although two fairly well controlled clinical trials in the early 1950s produced no evidence that DES was effective in this regard. Physicians continued to use DES until 1970 when it was discovered that, administered in the first trimester of pregnancy, it is teratogenic, often causing malformation of the internal genitalia of offspring, and sometimes precipitating a rare form of vaginal and cervical cancer in young females aged 7-25 (Herbst *et al.*, 1977). There is little evidence that DES prevented miscarriage.

In 1974, four years after the FDA ban, a prescription survey by the Health Research Group (1977) found 500,000 prescriptions for DES and similar hormones in treatment of pregnant women (Science News, 1977). Clearly, the confidence of a doctor in his own judgement of efficacy can be dangerous to his patients.

Psychotropic Drugs and Overprescribing

The phenomenon of overprescribing of psychotropic drugs illustrates a problem unit at large. Valium is the psychotropic drug most often prescribed in the US; Librium is the second. Both are benzodiazepines, minor tranquillisers, indicated for use in anxiety. Valium is often prescribed as a muscle relaxant. Parish (1974) reports that one-fifth of all prescriptions in England and Wales are for psychotropic drugs, and that Valium, Librium and Mogadon have made the greatest contribution to psychotropic drug increase in the decade 1961 to 1971.

Cooperstock (1974) cites a steady decline in the percentage of sedatives, hypnotics, and stimulants prescribed in England, Wales and Canada, but notes a rise in the percentage of tranquillisers and antidepressants. In 1970, 63 per cent of all tranquilliser prescriptions called for Librium or Valium.

Given that psychotropic drugs are widely prescribed, who are the major recipients? The sex of the patient is an important determinant. Women are prescribed psychotropics more than twice as often as men, although there is no evidence that women suffer more minor or major mental illness or psychological distress. There is a higher frequency of women's visits to physicians. Lennane and Lennane report that women are two to three times more likely to receive a psychotropic prescription for disorders which may have an organic base, such as dysmenorrhoea or nausea of pregnancy. This is particularly dangerous in the case of women who are or might be pregnant, since many seemingly innocuous drugs have been shown to be teratogenic, including aspirin, and the formerly 'safe' tranquilliser, thalidomide.

The use of drugs which affect the central nervous system during normal labour and delivery is almost as widespread in the US as medical participation in the normal birth process. Most drugs which suppress central nervous system functioning cross the placental barrier and can result in suppression of the baby's normal breathing response, slow its response to cold stress, and among other complications sometimes inhibit the newborn's behavioural response patterns up to a week after birth.

Many tranquillisers and analgesics slow up labour or cause it to cease entirely, requiring additional drug intervention with a labour stimulant, such as Poxytocin or Caesarian surgery. They may also adversely affect the neonate (Brazleton, 1970). Polypharmacy is the rule rather than the exception in normal birth despite the work by Lamaze, Leboyer and others showing excellent results in pain relief and participation by undrugged mothers in delivery.

The incidence of tranquilliser prescriptions increases with age for both sexes. As noted by Hemminki and Heikkil (1975) the institutionalised aged receive more drugs of all kinds including those acting on the central nervous system. Minor and major tranquillisers are widely used for easier patient management in psychiatric institutions and long-term care facilities as well. Sheppard *et al.* (1974) found polypharmacy, the use of several psychoactive drugs, to be a strong trend in psychiatric hospitals in the US.

A study of 47 general practitioners' prescribing habits (Hemminki, 1976) found that, on average, one drug was prescribed for each diagnosis, one in ten were psychotropic drugs, and one in 14 contained a 'hidden psychotropic' usually combined in one dosage form with a somatic drug. The prescribing frequencies varied greatly from doctor to doctor, correlating positively with the length of the physician's work day, and his attitude towards drug use to alleviate social problems and everyday stress. No correlation was found between estimated psychic disturbance patients and the rate of prescribing of psychotropic drugs. Similarly, Blum *et al.* (1972) found that physicians with a positive attitude toward drug use for recreation, and those who believed in the general ineffectiveness, mildness and benevolence of drugs, prescribed more psychotropics for their patients. They also recommended more OTC compounds and used more drugs themselves.

Those who considered medicine generally as more potent not only were less frequent self-medicators or prescribers, but also advocated stronger physical controls on narcotics' availability.

Advertising to Physicians

Silverman and Lee (1974) report that the FDA estimates that, in 1966, pharmaceutical firms spent about 600 million dollars in advertising, half of it on salaries and expenses for detail men, and with good reason: detail men are perceived by doctors to be the most acceptable form of advertising (Fassold and Gowley, 1968). That total advertising expenditure amounted to 3,000 dollars per physician for one year. The estimated figure for 1969 was 900 million spent for advertising, a 50 per cent increase. The ratio of detail men to medical practitioners varies greatly between countries (Hemminki and Personen, 1977). In the early 1970s, in Brazil and in Mexico, it was about 1 : 3 and 1 : 4; in the US, the United Kingdom and Finland it was between 1 : 14 and 1 : 18; and in Norway 1 : 32.

An average detail man visits a physician on his caseload about 50 times a year. Detail men provide physicians with useful clinical information, but their main goal, like all forms of advertising, is to 'sell the product'. In the US, the toxicity of chloramphenicol was played down until strict requirements were federally adopted. Hemminki (1977) has analysed the content of presentations to groups of doctors in Helsinki by detail men from 30 drug companies. She found that side effects and contraindications were often neglected. The drug presented was always recommended as the drug of choice; other forms of treatment were seldom mentioned.

In addition to advertising, drug companies often sponsor scholarships, grants and professional symposia devoted to new drugs or clinical problems in which their new drugs may be of value. Silverman and Lee (1974) charge that companies use these to introduce and promote their product under the guise of unbiased clinical reports of efficacy presented at the symposia, which are then picked up in reviews and reports to the medical community at large. Pharmaceutical houses also publish and distribute, free of charge, their own periodicals, similar in format to professional journals.

Professional journals themselves have the heaviest rate of advertising of all journals. The Journal of the American Medical Association grosses 7 million dollars a year from drug advertising; professional journals rarely review advertising content before publishing it. The FDA reviews unwarranted claims or misleading information in advertising of prescription drugs and may require manufacturers to withdraw advertisements or give public disclaimers and revisions.[3] In the absence of advertising standards enforced by disinterested parties, drug information so communicated is likely to be inadequate.

Advertising for psychotropic drugs bears certain unique characteristics. Between 30-40 per cent of drug advertising in medical journals is for psychotropic drugs, and two-thirds concern their use for what conventionally would be called non-medical indications, that is, emotional rather than physiological disorders, often portraying normal life stress, anger, and dissatisfaction as medically treatable afflictions (Stimson, 1975a).

Women are more often portrayed as suffering from emotional illness than somatic disorders and are more often the subject of advertisements for psychotropics than men, and have been portrayed only as patients, never as therapists, in spite of the fact that 15 per cent of psychiatrists are women (McCree *et al.*, 1974; Seidenberg, 1971). Forty-five per cent of the psychiatrists surveyed by McCree believed that the sexual bias in advertising might negatively influence physicians' perceptions of women, especially if the physicians lacked psychological training.

Smith (1977), performing a content analysis of the appeals used in psychotropic drug advertising, finds that these encourage at-a-glance diagnosis. Further, the physician is exposed to emotional appeals, i.e. 'non-rational', especially in the illustrations. The effects of such messages have not been evaluated, but certainly the advertisers, spending billions worldwide on such media, must presume their success.

Stimson's work on advertising is instructive. He finds (1975b, 1976a) that a typical English general practitioner receives about 35 free journals monthly and 50 mailed advertisements; the doctor will see at least one drug company detail man a week. The total number of individual advertisements (summing those within journals) is about 1,300 each month.

Examining how women were portrayed for contraceptive advertisements, they appear as young, efficient, well-groomed, idle and childless. They are shown as married, and Stimson characterises them as demure and confident. In contrast, the women in psychoactive drug advertisements — outnumbering men there by 15 to 1 — are portrayed as older, harassed, dishevelled,.with nagging children in tiresome settings.

That there is a stereotyped image presented to physicians with respect to female candidates for medicines is clear. In the materials Stimson analysed, the roles are of isolated and/or dependent creatures without 'a place of their own in society'. Smith's review (1977) further supports the presence of sex role stereotyping in advertisements.

With respect to the information contained in advertisements, Stimson examined promotional materials for general practitioners, (1976b), studying scientific referencing for claims; only 35 per cent of advertisements in periodicals offered evidence citations, although a subset analysed showed 2.6 references per piece of unique copy. Of these citations, over one-quarter were not available in libraries. Drug companies were themselves asked to supply the references and were able to do so for only 82 per cent of the citations.

With reference to information content, Stimson found (1975c, 1977) that advertisements to doctors do not provide sufficient facts relevant to prescribing. In addition to providing patient stereotypes (43 per cent of space) the actual content of advertisements pictures the product itself, (27 per cent of space), and pictures of diseases (9 per cent).

Smith (1977) has reviewed the literature on advertising reliance and impact. Although physicians claim to spend 19 minutes a day 'acquiring drug information', most evaluations of acquisition are based on self-appraisals rather than behaviour change tests.

Certainly the impact may not be as information-givers anticipate; more than a quarter of a group of doctors exposed to FDA warnings about a drug already in use disregarded side-effect information. Given the uncertainty as to impact, Smith concludes, as does Miller (1974), that a conclusion as to a major influence on prescribing by advertising is unwarranted, it may only be 'possibly effective'.

Does education of physicians help to counterbalance the influence of advertising? In an experimental series of courses in two Canadian universities, reported by Daniel and Leedham (1966), medical students were exposed to teachers with critical attitudes toward claims for new drugs in a programme designed to develop techniques for critical evaluation of these claims. Those students became significantly more sceptical than their unexposed colleagues, and remained so for a few years at least; no long-range follow-up was reported. Since Stolley *et al.* (1972) report that physicians with more postgraduate education tended to be better prescribers, it appears that attention should be given to continuing medical education for physicians, and possibly development of critical evaluation courses as described by Daniel and Leedham (1966) if one is to supplement clinical pharmacological training with the intent of improving prescription quality.

Certainly self-supervision for quality is not easily obtained. For example, Rosser (1975) reports on a national self-evaluation programme in Canada which provides ongoing information and self-evaluation forms by mail to busy physicians. The programme is promising and those who have used it seem quite satisfied; however, it is not widely used. Only a few doctors have shown an interest in its two years of operation, and physician participation on a continuing basis is extremely low.

Buchanan and Loxdal (1971) interviewed a sample of 66 Saskatchewan physicians about the ways they continued their education. First choice of method of 22 per cent was reading of medical journals, 20 per cent relied mainly on casual contacts with colleagues. Audio digests were preferred by 13 per cent, refresher courses by only 7 per cent, consultants 7 per cent; 15 per cent did not list any method for continuing their education. The researchers concluded that the problem was under or non-utilisation of existing resources by physicians. Personal obstacles, such as lack of time and organisation, fatigue and pressure, account or were at least rationalisations for 70 per cent of failures to keep up to date.

Similar findings have been reported by the Bureau of Research and Planning of the California Medical Association (1968) in a survey on continuing medical education for physicians. Most physicians reported getting information they needed by attending two- or three-day symposia, or reading journals and texts. But respondents frequently reported encountering difficulties in attending symposia, generally due to lack of time: 44-52 per cent of the respondents reported that they frequently found interesting programmes that they could not attend because of the time they would have to take away from their practice.

Hospital or university based drug information centres first established around 1962 have provided a potential resource for physicians in the US. The purposes they were initially designed to serve were broad and comprehensive. Although these services are available in many places throughout the US, their facilities are grossly under-utilised. Most physicians would not be willing to pay even 50 dollars a year for such services, and almost all the questions directed to drug information centres are technical usage questions, not consultation about choice of drugs or rational drug therapy. Significantly, drug information centres have not been cited as sources of drug information or continuing education by any physicians in the studies included here, in spite of the potential for contribution in the area.

Unavailability of accurate prescription data causes a problem with prescription review of private practitioners in countries without national health plans, and presents an obstacle to general prescription data collection. Rucker (1976) has proposed a computerised system for the US, where all prescribing would be handled through a data-bank from physician to pharmacist including communication and retrieval of information for billing or third-party payment, to official review of individual physicians and national drug consumption figures. Estimated cost would be 600 million dollars per year.

Czechoslovakia has a version of a computer system operating in four of Prague's ten districts; important differences exist there, however. Only about 1,000 different drugs are marketed and most of them manufactured in the country; all are distributed through a single national supplier. There is some question as to whether a computerised system would be cost effective and practical on as large a scale as Rucker proposes, especially in a free-market economy with a large population of heavy drug consumers and a vast number of chemical entities on the market.

It is apparent that the present methods for monitoring prescription practices and for improving physician competence are, at least in large and complex societies, inadequate. There is no lack of proposals for remedy, although none are of demonstrated cost effectiveness. A few can be listed: (1) For general supervision, pharmaceutical companies are required to make their sales figures available on a confidential basis to public agencies; these figures should be compared with disease prevalence data and clinical pharmacological standards so that trends in dubious practising can be noted early on. (2) The professionalisation (education, licensing) of detail men is required.[4] (3) Mandatory prescription peer review committees in all hospitals and as part of all health service supervisory mechanisms are desirable.[5] (4) Prescriptions of certain drugs to certified specialists should be limited. (5) Prescriptions of certain drugs should be limited to hospitalised patients or to those receiving a formal consultation prior to prescription. (6) Periodic reexamination of physicians' knowledge of clinical pharmacology is required. (7) Informed consent forms should be signed by patients receiving any medications classed as having a high risk of adverse effects. (8) Consumer education as to drug use should be expanded, encouraging patients to require information of their doctors and persuading patients to be quick to report untoward effects.

Generic Prescribing and Consumer Savings

The issue of generic prescription can well be considered under economics rather than in this chapter dealing with individual and social influences. If, however, it is assumed that the consumer is both knowledgeable and rational, seeking the same drug product at a lower price, then generic drug availability may be a factor in consumer decisions. Similarly, were it to be assumed that physicians were cost conscious, either on behalf of their patients or health service systems (governmental or private insurers), then the availability of cheaper versions of the same pharmaceuticals ought to be selected as part of the decision process. For that reason, generic drugs are considered here, even though one must acknowledge from the outset that economic models of rational decision-making based on low cost as a 'utility' leave much to be desired when it comes to explaining human behaviour.

Generic drugs come into existence as named products on the market after the patents of the original developers/manufacturers have expired. At that time, 17 years in the US, other producers can market the same drug, either under new trade names or under the generic name which is a common-usage term related to its chemical structural name.

Manufacturers producing patent-expired compounds may produce the same drug under two labels, a brand name and the generic name. Several manufacturers may produce the same compound competing under the same generic label. In that competition, both brand (trade, proprietary) and generic products may be offered at the prices the manufacturer wishes to set. That is not the case in controlled or licensed economies where governments set price and production policies.

There have been arguments about generic quality; it has been contended that generic equivalents may differ in absorption time and solubility as a function of manufacturing differences. That issue now seems moot; most studies find such differences minimal and conclude that generic products on the Western world markets do meet governmental pharmaceutical standards and, further, find that brand names and associated higher cost products do not assure better quality. In view of this and of lower pricing, many consumer organisations have taken the position that physicians should prescribe by generic name. The US Consumers Union advocates have so argued as has the European Public Health Committee Report on the Abuse of Medicines (1975).

Psychological factors, nevertheless, operate to influence the actual decisions made. Muller (1967) found that in New York City hospitals, the shorter proprietary (brand) names are more often selected for prescription, there being a significant correlation between short names and increased choice. A company first marketing a product which emerges with a short, 'catchy' name may thereby continue to command a market, by virtue of name appeal and habit, even after patents expire and competitive generic products appear.

Generic marketing as a legal concept would require that all drugs be marketed under generic names only; although the original manufacturer would retain his patent rights as sole producer of a new drug for a number of years, when the patent ran out he would not retain the advantage of a more familiar name for a generally available chemical compound. If a physician were convinced of one manufacturer's products' superiority, he or she could request the drug produced by that specific manufacturer. Azarnoff *et al.* (1966) point out that one danger in not prescribing generically is that brand-name drugs may be combination preparations and the single name conceals the contents; the physician could unknowingly duplicate contents in separate prescriptions to be consumed simultaneously.

Presently in the US, several States allow a pharmacist to substitute a generically marketed form of a drug, if available, for a brand-name form prescribed by the physician; if a physician prescribes a drug by its generic name, the pharmacist may sell any generically equivalent drug, whether it is marketed under a brand name or not.

This generic substitution may save the consumer money, providing the pharmacy has less expensive drugs in stock and passes its savings on to the consumer. Several studies have been conducted to determine how much money would be saved, under the present marketing system, through use of generic prescribing (or substitution by pharmacy).

Gumbhir and Rodowskas (1974) investigated the difference in cost between generic and brand name forms of seven drugs at 23 independent and 23 chain store pharmacies. They found that for 5 out of the 7 drugs at 45 of the 46 pharmacies, the generic form was cheaper than the brand-name version, and that some, but not all, of the savings to the pharmacy were passed on to the consumer.

Similarly, the Task Force on Prescription Drugs (1968) in investigating drug use among those over 65, found that generic prescription would save the elderly a considerable amount of money; assuming an average pharmacy mark-up, this would be an average of $1.10 per prescription on those drugs which are no longer under patent. Unfortunately, most drugs used by the elderly are still under patent and a few which are not can be purchased more cheaply under a brand name than generically.

In a study of 33 pharmacists in Rochester, New York, Horvitz and others (1975) found that out of 12 products, 4, including 2 widely used antibiotics, were often filled generically at a saving to the consumer, and 3 others were occasionally sold generically for substantially less than their brand-name counterparts. For the remaining 5 products, no savings were obtained when they were filled generically. Azarnoff *et al.* (1966) found that when Miltown was supplied generically as meprobamate at 17 pharmacies, an average saving of 17 per cent was realised. A separate survey showed that meprobamate from 10 different manufacturers all met USP standards, so a baseline for quality was somewhat assured.

Several factors must operate together in order for a consumer to save money with generically filled prescriptions. First, generically equivalent drugs must be available and marketed competitively. Second, the pharmacist must be aware of the existence of generic equivalents for many drugs, and must stock them and with a fair mark-up, pass on savings to the consumers. In States which prohibit generic substitution by pharmacists, this responsibility for awareness rests with the physician. Horvitz *et al.* (1975) found that pharmacists in their survey correctly identified out of 22 drugs, a mean of 18.5 as products for which other than brand-name products were available. A survey of physicians found that they correctly identified 14.1. Pharmacists who were better informed tended to stock and substitute low-cost generics for their patrons.

Jackson and Smith (1974) in a study of pharmacies in the southern US, report that there was no relationship between the cost of pre-scriptions and the quality of pharmaceutical services or the volume of prescriptions filled, and no relationship between the cost of one prescription and another. Smith (1976) suggested that the consumer is better off to shop for a family pharmacy with a good fee-to-service mix, and work with his pharmacist and his physician to achieve maximum savings.

Hospitals or health services can reduce purchasing costs and pass on savings to patients by bulk purchase of lower-priced generic drugs. Hospital formularies can provide a guide to rational prescribing as well as improving cost control; Muller found that 88 per cent of hospitals surveyed in New York State had up-to-date formularies but only about half limited doctors to prescribing from the formulary in the absence of special approval.

Furstenberg's study of a public medical care programme in Boston showed that with increased supervision, conformity to the formulary reached 70 per cent and other 20 per cent of prescribing was considered 'in the spirit of the formulary'.

When payment for drugs is made by a third party, restriction on reimbursement to drugs on a specified list has proven effective in altering prescribing. Studies have shown that, in general, prescribing habits among physicians remain considerably stable over time (Muller, 1967; Forsythe, 1963) so that a standard formulary with minor yearly revisions will remain up to date, making both bulk purchase and savings possible.

From all the indications, physicians generally underutilise this potential money-saving device of prescribing generically although they can be persuaded to do so if programmes are undertaken to educate them and to make generic prescribing easier. Quality of prescribing can also be influenced by formularies. Evidently, there is a need for both. Lilja (1976) in Sweden reports a study of prescribing appropriateness indicating that, taking both medical and economic aspects into account, 65 per cent of the physicians made unsatisfactory choices of drugs in cases of bacterial pneumonia.

Hospital pharmacists providing clinical pharmacy services may be able to effect savings for patients. Ryan *et al.* (1975) showed the effect of 'discharge interviews' of 1,000 patients in a university hospital. Pharmacists worked with physicians to substitute less expensive drugs when possible, to secure third-party payment coverage for those eligible, and recommend purchase of OTC remedies where appropriate.

The result of the exercise was that savings of nearly $1,700 were realised on 517 out of 1,832 prescriptions, about $9.13 per hour of pharmacist time. Smith has suggested that pharmacist-physician co-operation outside the hospital can similarly reduce drug cost to the consumer and may improve outpatient prescribing.

The Personal Context of Use of Medicine

Assumption and Evidence

Most of the research which has been cited in the previous sections of this chapter has been based on commonly held assumptions about the role of the health care system in society and the participation of the public in that system. Recently, these assumptions have been challenged by many observers in the field, among them Zola (1973); Pratt (1976); Mechanic (1976); McKeown (1976); Dubois (1959); and Illich (1976). The following is a critical analysis of some underlying assumptions.

Assumption: When People are Ill, they Normally Consult a Physician.
After reviewing data from medical care studies from the US and Great Britain, White *et al.* (1961) reported that for two-thirds of all episodes of illness, physicians were not consulted. Zola (1972) estimates the figures to be closer to nine out of 10 illnesses which were not reported to physicians; these figures reflect serious as well as minor medical problems.

This is an area where a number of parallel studies could be conducted in a wide variety of countries for comparative purposes. Such studies should be rather easy to carry out in developing as well as developed countries since they do not require for their accomplishment any sophisticated equipment. A short standardised questionnaire, which could be easily turned into a standardised interview, would be all the apparatus needed, in addition to a modest number of health workers with minimum training for simple field work.

It would be interesting to uncover what is universal and what is culturally determined in the selection of illnesses or phases of illnesses (or syndromes) concerning which physicians are usually consulted. Such information should be significantly valuable for developers of health service programmes, tailor-made to suit various cultural settings. Relevant here are some proverbs still considered invaluable by certain sectors of Egyptian society. Following are but two examples: (1) consult an experienced man rather than a doctor; (2) live by wisdom and you are always sick (note, one of the many connotations of the Arabic word for wisdom is medical expertise) (Soueif, 1978).

Wadsworth *et al.* (1971) found that perceived ill health, rather than actual illness, determines in part who seeks medical help. The individual's interpretation of his symptoms determines when and whether they will be brought to a physician's attention. If a complaint were familiar, or shared by members of the individual's social group or occupation, and the course of the disorder was known, it was less likely that the individual would seek medical attention. Zola (1973) found that when people sought medical help for symptoms they had had for some time, the precipitating factor for seeking help was not related to worsening of symptoms; unrelated psychological stress or discovery that the symptom interfered with work or play were often motivating factors.

In the Blums' (1965) study of health practices in rural Greece, it was observed that peasants considered it normal and desirable for their children to contract the usual communicable childhood diseases. They did not seek medical help, nor restrict the children's activities while they were ill since they viewed the illness as part of the normal course of events.

In Egypt more or less similar practices are to be noted. In a number of rural districts the family will not seek medical help so long as the disease is perceived as part of the normal course of the child's life events. In many cases, the family would encourage the 'not-yet-fallen-ill child' to mix with the diseased sibling so that he or she would get the infection (e.g. measles) and pass through what is perceived as a stage in a normal course of development (Soueif, 1978).

Greenley and Mechanic (Mechanic, 1976) found that socio-cultural variables affect the individual's decision to seek medical help, independent of the discomfort or stress produced by the illness. A more extreme example occurs in the Canadian work of the Cummings (1957). In an effort to improve mental health, these psychiatrists, working on one town, sought to teach citizens major psychiatric diagnoses, explaining for example, how people who hallucinated and were otherwise out of contact were not, as their families thought, merely 'eccentric' but were schizophrenic. Under the folk definition of eccentricity these people were accepted and cared for at home. Under the new mental health approach, they were clearly psychotic and must be treated medically, at that time in hospital. Townpeople resisted education which turned the familiar into the frightening and would have made family members into inpatients in hospitals, which townsfolk knew to be thoroughly unpleasant places. The investigators, honestly confronting their errors and angry citizens, left town. Folk diagnoses had, for understandable reasons, won out.

Easy access to free or low-cost medical care does not seem to alter this phenomenon of the dominance of folk-founded definitions of health and illness. A related assumption involves people's utilisation of preventive health care measures. One presumes that preventive services, when available, will be utilised. A notable example is found in the 1958 polio vaccination programme in the US. A favourable attitude on the part of a mother did not ensure vaccination of her children. In one study, 46 per cent of the children whose mothers had favourable attitudes were not vaccinated, sometimes due to inappropriate beliefs, that the children were not highly susceptible to the disease, but more often, due to 'plain procrastination', the absence of a specific motivating force to get the child vaccinated (Glasser, 1958). Most significantly, findings by both Glasser (1958) and Merrill *et al.* (1958) indicated that people tended to behave the way they thought their friends and neighbours behaved in spite of the medical information available to the public.

The generality of this resistance to attention is emphasised by Morris (1957) who examined disease prevalence for those at varying levels of illness, risk, medical care experience, and readiness to use medical services (when free, as in the UK). The populations at higher illness risk, or with more actual morbidity, were those least disposed to seek medical care. One assumes here that some of the same education, class and personality factors which increase risk are also associated with increasing isolation from the knowledge system which is medicine in practice.

Assumption: When People Report their Symptoms to their Physician, he makes an Accurate Diagnosis and Prescribes Drugs Solely on the Basis of that Diagnosis. The way that symptoms are reported to the physician depends in part on cultural background and may influence prescribing. In Zola's (1973) study of illness reporting among cultural groups in America, he found that for the same disorder, Irish Catholics did not report pain, but a difficulty in accomplishing tasks, while Italian Catholics described diffuse, painful symptoms. The latter group received more prescriptions, unrelated to the medical severity of the disease. Cartwright (1974) reports on her study of elderly British patients; she discovered that most patients had arrived at a self-diagnosis before they saw the doctor. They tended to present only those symptoms they felt the doctor could treat and presented them in a way they thought would be acceptable to him. Cartwright also found that almost uniformly, patients who expected drugs received them, even if the medicine was a placebo. Fewer prescriptions were given to the patient when the physician found him 'easy to talk to', more when the doctor found the consultation less satisfactory.

Freidson (1961) describes the history of a complaint as first, self-diagnosis, followed by consultation with members of the patient's family or friends for confirmation or alteration. Self-treatment usually follows, and if the complaint persists, a doctor may be consulted for diagnosis and treatment. Lay consultation continues throughout this phase. Freidson observes:

> Interaction with non-professional consultants in the lay referral structure is just as responsible for the patients not following the doctor's orders or not returning for further treatment as are cessation of symptoms and the patient's personal opinions about proper treatment. Obviously relevant are the norms surrounding the sick role, the conception of illness, its causes and cures, and norms surrounding the consultant's role.

A study by Balint *et al.* (1970) also shows evidence of the influence of patient desires on prescribing. The investigators conclude that most repeat prescriptions, which are not strictly appropriate medical treatment, are a diagnosis of a deficient doctor-patient relationship, where the physician and patient tacitly agree not to admit to close examination of the patient's life problems and needs. Whether it is for a psychoactive, a somatic or a placebo drug, the prescription provides a substitute for 'something that the patient needs from his environment' and is usually demanded by the patient as a condition for a peaceful, mutually appreciative relationship with the physician.

Balint *et al.* characterise the typical repeat prescription patients as desiring but avoiding intimacy: most patients tended to telephone for the refill prescription, send for it via a third party, or make a brief visit to the physician's office marked by impersonal conversation and the absence of a physical examination. If a patient tried to break this pattern he had initiated, by suggesting he no longer was in need of the medicine, the physician generally opposed the move, presumably for fear of upsetting a fragile, satisfactory relationship. Physicians who were more comfortable admitting hostility and dissatisfaction toward their patients and had an easier time accepting those feelings from patients tended to give fewer repeat prescriptions.

Mechanic (1976) found that a physician who saw more patients was more apt to describe patient complaints as trivial or inappropriate. He reports that many factors affect physician behaviour, including social orientation, patient demands, degree of bureaucratic organisation of practice setting and physician attitudes towards the work ethic.

Correct diagnosis is considered a prerequisite to appropriate drug use; yet Duff and Hollingshead (1968) reported that over half of the cases in their hospital study had been misdiagnosed. In several large series of autopsies the antemortem diagnoses were found to be wrong in 40-50 per cent of patients (Prutting, 1978). And Brook *et al.* (1976) in their review write, 'in the last 60 years, nearly 1,000 studies have been done to assess the level of quality of care delivered . . . Virtually all of these studies have detected basic problems in the level of quality delivered'.

Assumption: The Most Appropriate and Desirable Model of the Physician-Patient Relationship is that of a Physician (Expert) Authority Figure and a Compliant (Passive) Patient. Patients Obey the Physician's Orders and get Well. This implied formulation of the doctor-patient relationship can be injurious to both parties, in practice. Blum (1960) reports that the patient who seeks an authoritarian physician, and relinquishes responsibility to the doctor is more likely to sue for malpractice. The more the gratitude, the greater the risk of disappointment. And the physician who accepts the role of authoritarian-protector is more likely, when things go wrong medically, to be inept in handling the relationship and be sued.

It may also be inimical to good health. Pratt (1976) (p. 189) found that the assumption that 'the physician's dominance is functional for therapy and that submissiveness is the ill person's appropriate response . . . is not supported by the findings, for submissiveness . . . produced poor health service for the patients'. Families which performed health care activities effectively, tended to foster individuality and independence in their members and to assert the members' interests in encounters with the health care system. Aspects of the system interfere with the patient's recovery and reassimilation into the healthy world insofar as they inhibit a family's ability to care for a sick member; restrictive hospital visiting rules are one example of this (Pratt, 1976).

Glogow (1973) found that health care professionals characterised the good patient as co-operative, helpful, happy, tidy and uncomplaining; in other words, easy for the staff to take care of. The 'bad patient' was described as unco-operative, noisy, belligerent, complaining and demanding; assertive and in an unpleasant way a 'crock'. Dunbar (1947) found that hospitalised tuberculosis patients described the 'good patient' much the same way as hospital administrators did. But he reported that the patients who conformed to this image of 'model patient' were the ones most likely to die or return later more seriously ill.

The 'bad patients' who displayed hostility and aggressiveness openly tended to recover more quickly and permanently − findings supported by other work in the field (Calden *et al.*, 1960; Daniels and Davidoff, 1950). Glogow (1973) has proposed that the issue is one of patient power. Good patients relinquish their power; bad patients, who retain a sense of power, exercise it toward their own recovery.

Janis (1958) in a study of reactions of patients to surgery found that those who were least anxious before surgery were more at risk of emotional disturbance afterwards. The quiet, 'good' patients were likely to be repressing their fears which, not then communicated to the physician, exploded afterwards when confronted with pain, physical constraint, and mutilation. Janis proposed 'psychological inoculation', the confrontation before surgery designed to ventilate feelings and to increase patient security by accurate predictions, on the part of the physician, as to what to expect.

Medical approval of the grateful, quiet, obedient consumer as the 'good patient' is unwise. People must take the health initiative in their own care. Individuals generally self-diagnose their condition, often consulting with other lay people for advice, self-medicate before they see a physician and often continue self-help and consultation while under professional care (Freidson, 1961).

Wadsworth *et al.* (1971) found that two-thirds of the medicines consumed by people in their study population were consumed on their own or another lay person's initiative. Ten out of the 15 most common disorders (ISC categories) were most often found and diagnosed by a lay person before being diagnosed by a physician. And lay diagnosis is not eradicated by free and available medical care (Wadsworth, 1971).

Another, more recent manifestation of patient assertiveness is doctor-shopping. People who are dissatisfied with some aspect of care will shop for another physician rather than suffer what they find to be objectionable conditions. Kasteler *et al.* (1976) discovered that

48 per cent of upper income families and 37 per cent of lower income families in the sample had changed physicians within a year prior to the interview. In both groups, major factors in the decision were a lack of confidence in their doctor's competence, their physician's unwillingness to spend time talking with patients, high cost of services, inconvenience of location and hours, and hostility toward doctors or unfavourable attitudes toward a doctor's personal qualities.

Previous studies in the US (Cahal, 1962) and England (Gray and Cartwright, 1953) had found that only 8 per cent and 10 per cent of the populations respectively, had changed doctors due to dissatisfaction. In the UK, however, administration factors make changing doctors difficult.

Assumption: Humans conform to the Rational Consensus. They will act as economic utilitarians, buying that which is effective, safe and cheap. They will respond to information that affects their self-interest by altering their conduct. Education of physicians will lead to improvement in their prescribing habits; information to consumers will lead to wiser use of medicines.

Sometimes, only sometimes. We shall not repeat citation of the studies which litter this chapter with evidence for consumers' non-response to information, to physician non-use of and non-response to education, or to the failure of that rational democratic device, the informed consent. The failures are only partial, for the studies also suggest that information is important, that education sometimes works, that there is a general correlation between communication, comprehension, satisfaction and consensus between physician and patient and proper drug use.

A rational medicines policy need not then be one which counts on giving information as the keystone to consumer health and economic well-being. A rational medicines policy more likely is one which takes into account as much as a person can learn about the determinants of health behaviour, prescription practices and medicine use.

Assumption: Major Inroads have been made in Eradicating Disease among the Human Population; Disease is Ultimately Conquerable through Surgery and Drugs. Success only Requires that Patients Visit the Doctor and do what he Says. Strides in medicine in the last forty years have made treatable a host of formerly life-threatening diseases, and in parts of the world vaccines have made epidemics of smallpox, typhoid and polio a thing of the past. These are selective, though substantial contributions. Wadsworth *et al.* (1974) presented two related principles: the Iceberg concept and the Onion principle. The former states that at any time diseases reported to the medical establishment only constitute the 'tip of the iceberg' — a greater proportion of cases lie beneath the surface and remain untreated. The latter states that when some major class of disease is eradicated, the underlying ones are revealed and take their place in importance; when infectious disease epidemics no longer take the lives of a substantial part of the population, cancer and heart disease become the killers.

And Butterfield (1968), who discovered that a majority of cases of diabetes in the study population remained unseen and untreated by 'available' medical services, found that many untreated cases were clinically very different from the cases seen by physicians. All in all, Dubos' characterisation of *The Mirage of Health* (1959) and McKeown's (1976) admonition to regard the limited scope of therapeutic interaction must be borne in mind; 'the determinants of health are largely outside the medical care system'.

One does not wish to extol therapeutic nihilism; medical advances have been marvellous. Nevertheless, one must recognise limits, these sometimes hidden behind undue faith in technological innovation. Consider that with the most expensive developments in acute cardiac care, the life span of treated versus untreated patients is greater for only 5 per cent of the treated over the untreated. Or consider, that for all its trauma, radical mastectomies now show no greater success rate than simple mastectomies over a follow-up period.

This is not to deny advances in cancer or cardiovascular therapy; it is to note that intervention does not equal success, and to be reminded, *à la* Dubos, that the major health improvements come about through changes in the environment and in life styles, including self-care, nutrition, safety, pollution control and sanitation and the like.

For medicines, the field is not yet clearly enough surveyed for one to be sure what conduct is entirely determined by external forces, i.e. drug availability, cost, medical indication or physician prescribing conduct as opposed to those variables which are grist for the social scientists' mill, that is, the economic, social and psychological features. It does appear, on the basis of the rather narrow evidence offered here, that much of what patients/consumers do rests on personal, folk, situational factors. Certainly that is demonstrated in the most intensively studied field of compliance. If so, then health and economic well-being do rest on the consumer's own decision, including those of whether to go to or co-operate with a doctor.

That being so, then it behoves those interested in the consumers' well-being to pay due regard to the events that affect them most; learning of these through research, working with these in experimental programmes, respecting them as salient forces in important human conduct. Certainly no public health effort can fail to focus on the importance of pharmacotherapeutics. Likewise, no broad concern with medicines policy can fail to address consumer behaviour, folk definitions of illness and health, the doctor-patient interaction which affects patient satisfaction and subsequent compliance, the personal and demographic features which influence that doctor-patient relationship as well as other health conduct and the family and friendship support networks which decide what is medicine and when and how it is to be used.

Final Comments

The scientific literature on factors influencing the use of medicines by individuals is limited to technologically advanced countries, and to populations with access to medicines and physicians in less advanced nations. There are but few studies with data to assist our understanding of medicine use by populations who rely entirely on folk medicine or manufactured pharmaceuticals, dispensed without qualified medical or pharmacist advice.

The data which is extant, much of it dubious because of poor research quality, suggests that:

(1) Even in advanced nations, much of what physicians define as illness goes unseen by physicians, but is self-treated through home remedies and self- or family-guided drug purchases. Many of these remedies may be ineffective; some are palliatives, some may be 'curative'. The factors which influence the choice of these remedies are primarily matters of folk culture. Essential to these are personal and family definitions of health and illness.

As with health *per se*, much medicine use is beyond the direct influence of medical care systems or health providers. This is obvious in prescription compliance as well as in self-medication or folk healing. Experts may define the use of medicines as a public health domain, but it is, in fact, a personal, family and peer affair. Insofar as medicines use is externally affected, it is regulatory policy or economics more than medical admonitions which will be dominant.

(2) While economic waste is evident and some toxic outcomes are observed, there is no evidence for great threats to public health from existing patterns of self-medication. The significant exceptions are in the cases of drugs of 'abuse', i.e. alcohol and tobacco or opiates which are used in a fashion contrary to already existing consumer wisdom and folk norms.

(3) Much of what physicians do by way of pharmacotherapeutics fails to conform to present standards of high quality care. Over-prescribing appears to be the most egregious error; diagnostic failure with prescription error is common. If one requires as a standard of care, sophistication about patients as people (e.g. knowledge of the correlates of common behaviours such as non-compliance, say the relationship of dissatisfaction and non-compliance to doctor behaviour and information-giving), then the majority of physicians, especially those engaged in treating ambulatory patients, seem inadequately informed. An unknown, but undoubtedly large, number then perform inadequately in prescribing.

(4) Education and information do have an impact on both physician and patient/consumer, but these influences are exaggerated as 'cures' for the various problems in medicine prescription or use. The concept of the rational man or woman, be that doctor or patient, has limited, albeit important, applicability. Thus, the efficacy of information cannot be assumed, although there is no evidence as yet as to 'dangerous side effects' from being informed – contrary to the convictions of more paternalistic practitioners. One cannot, however, rule out anxiety as a consequence of information and as a subsequent disruptor of behaviour. On the other hand, that same anxiety can be helpful as a stimulus to action, if social supports and clear directions for appropriate action exist to channel it.

(5) Given numerous failures in programmes designed to recruit patients to medical care, to produce better compliance, to enhance medical care quality, to reduce unwise drug use, it is apparent that programmes for voluntary change involving significant resources or expectations should not be undertaken without prior research, including field

evaluations of pilot or test programmes. There will be circumstances in which public health can be rather quickly assisted by policies which do not rely on voluntary behaviour, as for example, regulations which remove or restrict access to hazards. Such controls may themselves have negative aspects so that here, too, cost/benefit estimates, pre-testing, and a salutory reading of history are in order.

(6) In policy and consumer literature, much emphasis is placed on economic forces. Their prominence is much more pronounced on the part of interest groups seeking to influence individuals than within the hierarchy of factors identified as salient for individuals themselves. Thus, the profit motive on the part of advertisers, economic considerations on the part of governments or labour force productivity interests can be strong forces seeking to affect what the medicine user does. On the other hand, the individual seems relatively indifferent to economic self-interest, getting best buys, avoiding useless products, insisting on generic drugs when it comes to accounting for what she (for more drugs buyers, users, and family healers are women) does with regard to the choice and use of medicines. This observation of minimal economic influence is, no doubt, restricted to ceilings on costs and purchases, these being implicit in family budgets or built in by health insurance or medicine cost control policies of health services.

(7) The literature on medicines' use cited here does not compel conclusions leading to medicines policies nor related social action. Such proposals as are commonly made derive from convictions based on more general opinions, as for example, those dealing with medical care quality, epidemiology, resource thrift or other economic ideology or morals, for example, those which may condemn advertising for being self-interested persuasion rather than scientific education for physicians and consumers.

Perhaps the lack of consensus either about problems or directions may be attributable to the generally limited or poor quality of research, to the demonstrated complexity of human health/medicines behaviour or to a current awareness that the prediction of the effects of programmed change is rather less easy than one — as either idealist, clinician or scientist — had initially anticipated.

There are, of course, numerous proposals for medicines policies designed to influence individual conduct, for example, those advocating consumer education, closer scrutiny of physician prescribing, controls over advertising, greater availability of generic drugs, improved pharmacology teaching for physicians, greater regulation of access to drugs, training physicians in relationship management and communication to patients, or creating in consumers a new role concept of the patient as a decision-making partner in treatment. These and other proposals are each reasonable, yet none are incontrovertibly proved as both necessary and cost effective.

Notes

1. According to the US Task Force on Prescription Drugs the elderly, on the whole, receive three times the number of prescriptions than those under 65, throughout the socioeconomic spectrum, receive. Elderly women, like their younger counterparts, use an average of 50 per cent more prescription medication than men of the same age group. A conference report on Drug Use and the Elderly (sponsored by the National Institute on Drug Abuse and the National Institute for Drug Programs) states that senior citizens in nursing homes average 300 dollars in drug bills every year, compared to 87 dollars for those who are not institutionalised. Part of this difference may reflect a greater rate of morbidity in the former group of persons, but 40 per cent of the drugs used act on the central nervous system: pain killers, sedatives and tranquillisers. Many prescriptions appear to be for easier patient management, not medical indications, and are used as a substitute for activities and involvement.

2. During 1966-8, when required to by the FDA, US companies altered their chloramphenicol labelling but the same companies continued 'misbranding' in the European market. On the other hand, following the publication of Silverman's book, advertisers appear to have voluntarily moved toward more factual labelling including warnings.

3. The FDA can preclear prescription advertisements when voluntarily requested to do so.

4. Some are pharmacists; some hold school certificates.

5. Therapeutic committees exist in hospitals; the quality of their supervision varies widely.

References

Azarnoff, D, *et al.* (1966). Prescription writing by generic name and drug cost. *Journal Clinical Pharmacology*

Bakker, C.B. and Dightman, C.R. (1964). Psychological factors in fertility control. *Fertility and Sterility 15*, 559

Balint, M. (1957). *The Doctor, His Patient and the Illness*, New York, International Universities Press

Balint, M. *et al.* (1970). *Treatment or Diagnosis: A Study of Repeat Prescriptions in General Practice*, Philadelphia, Tavistock Publications, J.B. Lippincott Co

Becker, M. *et al.* (1972). Predicting mother's compliance with pediatric medical regimens. *Journal Pediatrics 81*, 843

Becker, M.H. *et al.* (1971). Characteristics and attitudes of physicians associated with prescribing of chloramphenicol. *HSMHA Health Reports 86*, 993

Becker, M.H. (1976). Facts of compliance: strategies for improvement. *Drug Therapy*, February

Becker, M.H. and Green, L.W. (1972). A family approach to compliance with medical treatment: a selective review of the literature. *International Journal of Health Education 18*, 131, 173

Becker, M. and Maiman, L. (1975). Sociobehavioral determinants of compliance with medical care recommendations. In *Medical Care 13*, 1, January

Blum, E. (1958). The uncooperative patient: the development of a test to predict uncooperativeness in medical treatment. In *Supplementary Studies on Malpractice*, San Francisco, Cal Medical Association

Blum, R. (1956). *A Study of Public Response to Disaster Warnings*, Stanford Research Institute, June

—— (1957). *The Psychology of Malpractice Suits*, California Medical Association

—— (1958). *Hospitals and Patient Dissatisfaction: A Study of Factors Associated with Malpractice Rates in Hospitals*, California Medical Association

—— (1960). Management of the doctor-patient relationship, New York, McGraw Hill

—— (1969). *Commonsense Guide to Doctors, Hospitals and Medical Care*, New York, Macmillan Co

Blum, R. *et al.* (1972). *The Dream Sellers*, San Francisco, Jossey-Bass Inc

Blum, R. and Blum, E. (1965). *Health and Healing in Rural Greece*, Stanford, California, Stanford University Press

Blum, R., Blum, E. and Garfield, E. (1976). *Drug Education: Results and Recommendations*, Lexington, Mass., D.C. Heath and Company

Bonner, J., Goldberg, A. and Smith, J.A. (1969). Do pregnant women take their iron? *Lancet 1*, 457

Boyd, J. *et al.* (1979). Drug defaulting, part II: analysis of noncompliance patterns. *American Journal of Hospital Pharm. 31*, 485-91, May

Brazelton, T.B. (1970). Effect of prenatal drugs on the behavior of the neonate. *American Journal of Psychiatry 126*, 95-100

Breault, H.J. (1979). Five years with five million child resistant containers. *Clinical Toxicol 7*, 91

Brodie, D. (1970). *Drug Utilization and Drug Utilization Review and Control*, Department of HEW-PHS-HSMHA-NCHSRD. April

Brook, R.H., Williams, K.N. and Avery, A.D. (1976). Quality assurance today and tomorrow: forecast for the future. *Annals of Internal Medicine 85*, 6, December

Buchanan, K. and Loxdal, O.E. (1971). Continuing education habits of Saskatchewan general practitioners. *CMA Journal 105*, December 18

Bureau of Research and Planning, California Medical Association (1968). A survey of continuing medical education for physicians. *California Medicine 109*, September

Bush, P.J. and Rabin, D.L. (1976). Who's using nonprescribed medicines? *Medical Care 14*, 12, December

Butterfield, W.J.H. (1968). *Priorities in Medicine*, The Nuffield Provincial Hospitals Trust

Butt, H.R. (1977). A method for better physician-patient communication. *Annals of Internal Medicine 86*, 478-80

Cahal, M.F. (1962). What the public thinks of the family doctor: folklore and facts. *GP 25*, 146-57

Calden, G., Dupertus, C.W., Hokanson, J.E. and Lewis, W.C. (1960). Psychosomatic factors in the rate of recovery from tuberculosis. *Psychosomatic Medicine 22*, 345-55, Sept-October

Cartwright, A. (1979). Prescribing and the relationship between patients and doctors. In *Social Aspects of Medical Use of Psychotropic Drugs*, Cooperstock, R. (Ed.), Addiction Foundation of Ontario

Charney, E. *et al.* (1967). How well do patients take oral penicillin? *Pediatrics 40*, 188

Christopher, L. and Crooks, J. (1979). Are we overconsuming? *World Health*, April

Clinite, J. and Kabat, H. (1976). Improving patient compliance. *Journal American Pharm. Association 16*, February

Cohen, M.N. (1976). *What Drug Information Should the Consumer Have? A Consumer Perspective*, San Francisco, Hastings College of Law, June 1976

Cole, P. and Emmanuel, S. (1971). Drug consultation: its significance for the discharged hospital patient and relevance as a role for the pharmacist. *American Journal of Hospital Pharm. 28*, December

Coleman, J.S., Katz, E. and Menzel, H. (1966). *Medical Innovation: A Diffusion Study*, Indianapolis, Bobbs Merrill

Cooperstock, R. (1979). Some factors involved in the increased prescribing of psychotropic drugs. In *Social Aspects of Medical Use of Psychotropic Drugs*, Cooperstock (ed.), Addiction Reserch Foundation of Ontario

Cummings, J. and Cummings, E. (1957). *Closed Ranks: An Experiment in Mental Education*, Cambridge, Mass., Harvard University Press

Daniel, E. and Leedham, L. (1966). Effect on student attitudes of a program of critical evaluation of claims for drugs. *Journal of Medical Education 41*, 49 January

Daniels, G.E. and Davidoff, E. (1950). The mental aspects of TB. *American Review of Tuberculosis 62, 5*: 532-38

Davis, M.S. (1968). Physiologic, psychological and demographic factors in patient compliance with doctor's orders. *Medical Care 6*, 115

—— (1968). Variations in patients' compliance with doctors' advice: an empirical analysis of patterns of communication. *American Journal of Public Health 58*, 274-88

Drug and Therapeutics Bulletin (1972). *10*, 25, December 8

Dubos, R. (1959). *The Mirage of Health*, New York, Harper Brothers

Duff, R.S. and Hollingshead, A.B. (1968). *Sickness and Society*, New York, Harper and Row

Dunbar, F. (1947). *Mind and Body: Psychosomatic Medicine*, New York, Random House.

Dunne, M., Herxheimer, A., Newman, M. and Ridley, H. (1973). Indications and warnings about chloramphenicol. *The Lancet 2*, 781-3

Dunnell, K. and Cartwright, A. (1972). *Medicine Takers, Prescribers and Hoarders*, London, Routledge and Kegan Paul

European Public Health Committee, Council of Europe (1975). *Abuse of Medicines, Part II: Prescription Medicines*

Farquhar and Maccoby (1975). Communications for health: unselling heart disease. *Journal of Communications 25*, 3, Summer

Fassold, R.W. and Gowley, C.W. (1968). A survey of physicians' reactions to drug promotion. *Canadian Medical Assoc. Journal 98*, 701, April 6

Fink, D.L. (1976). Tailoring the consensual regimen. In Sackett, D. and Haynes, R.H. *Compliance with Therapeutic Regimens*, Baltimore, Johns Hopkins University Press

Fleckenstein, L. (1976). Attitudes of users towards oral contraceptives information. In Lasagna, *Patient Compliance*, New York, Futura, Mt. Kisko

Forsythe, G. (1963). An enquiry into the drug bill. *Medical Care 1*, 1 January-March

Francis, V. *et al.* (1969). Gaps in doctor patient communication: patient response to medical advice. *New England Journal of Medicine 280*, 535

Freidson, E. (1961). *Patients Views of Medical Practice*, New York, Russell Sage Foundation

Garrettson, L.K. (1977). The child resistant container: a success and a model for accident prevention. *AJPH 67*(2), 135, February

Garner, D.D. (1971). Study of drug utilization patterns through prescription analysis. PhD Dissertation, University of Miss

Glasser, M.A. (1958). A study of the public's acceptance of the Salk vaccine program. *AJPH 48*, 141, February

Glogow, E. (1973). The 'bad patient' gets better quicker. *Social Policy 4*, November/December

Gray, P.G. and Cartwright, A. (1953). Choosing and changing doctors. *The Lancet*, 1308-9

Green, L.W. (1977). Evaluation and measurement: some dilemmas for health education. *American Journal of Public Health 67*, 2, February

Greenley, J.R. and Mechanic, D. (1976). The prevalence of psychological distress and help-seeking in a college student population. *Social Psychiatry 11*, (1), January, 1-14

Gumbhir, A. and Rodowskas, C. (1974). Consumer price differentials between generic and brand name prescriptions. *American Journal Public Health 64*, 10, October, 977

Hammond, E.C. (1963). The influence of health on smoking habits. Presented at the Statistics Section Meeting of the American Public Health Association, Kansas City, November 13

Hassar, M. and Weintraub, M. (1976). Uninformed consent and the healthy volunteer: an analysis of patient volunteers. In 'A clinical trial of a new anti-inflammatory drug', *Clinical Pharmacology and Therapeutics 20*, 4, October

Haynes, R. (1976). Critical review of the determinants of patient compliance with therapeutic regimens. In Sackett and Haynes, *Compliance with Therapeutic Regimens*, Baltimore, Johns Hopkins University Press

—— (1976). Strategies for improving compliance: a methodological analysis and review. In Sackett and Haynes, *Compliance with Therapeutic Regimens*, Balitmore, Johns Hopkins University Press

Heinzelmann, F. and Bagley, R.W. (1970). Response to physical activity programs and their effects on health behavior. *Public Health Rep. 85*, 905

Hemminki, E. and Heikkil, A. (1975). Elderly people's compliance with precriptions, and quality of medication. *Scandinavian Journal Social Medicine 3* (2), 87-92

—— (1976). Factors influencing drug prescribing: an inquiry into research strategy. *Drug Intelligence and Clin. Pharm. 10*, June

—— (1977). Content analysis of drug-detailing by pharmaceutical representatives. *Medical Education 2*, 210-15

Hemminki, E. and Personen, T. (1977). The function of drug company representatives. *Scandinavian Journal of Soc. Med. 5*, 105-14

Herbst, A.L., Cole, P., Colton, T., Robboy, S.J. and Scully, R.E. (1977). Age-incidence and risk of diethylstilbestrol-related clear cell adenocarcinoma of the vagina and cervix. *American Journal of Obstetrics and Gynecology 128*, May 1, 43

Hermann, F. (1973). The outpatient prescription label as a source of medication errors. *American Journal of Hospital Pharm. 30*, Feb., 155

Herxheimer, A. (1977). L'Automedication. In *Thérapeutique Médicale*, Febre, J. *et al.*, Paris, Flammarion

Hladik, W.B. III and White, S.J. (1976). Evaluation of written reinforcements used in counseling cardiovascular patients. *American Journal Hospital Pharm. 33*, December, 1277-80

Horvitz, R.A., Morgan, J.P. and Fleckenstein, L. (1975). Savings from generic prescriptions: a study of 33 pharmacies in Rochester, New York. *Ann. Intern. Med. 82* (5) May, 601-7

Hulka, B. *et al.* (1976). Communication, compliance and concordance between physicians and patients with prescribed medications. *American Journal Public Health 66*, 9

Illich, I. (1976). *Medical Nemesis*, New York, Pantheon Press

Jackson, R. and Smith, M. (1974) Relations between price and quantity in community pharmacy. *Medical Care 12*, 1 January

Janis, L. (1958). *Psychological Stress*, New York, John Wiley and Sons

Johannsen, W.J. *et al.* (1966). On accepting medical recommendations. *Arch. Environ. Health 12*, 63

Johnson, R.E., Pope, C.R., Campbell, W.H. and Azevedo, D.J. (1976). Reported use of nonprescribed drugs in health maintenance. *Am. J. Hosp. Pharm. 33*, December 1249-54

Joyce, C.R.B. *et al.* (1968). Personal factors as a cause of differences in prescribing by general practitioners. *British Journal Prev. Social Medicine 22*, 170

Julian, P. and Herxheimer, A. (1977). Doctors' anxieties in prescribing. Reprint from *Journal of the Royal College of General Practitioners 27*, 662-5

Kasteler, J. *et al.* (1976). Issues underlying prevalence of doctor shopping behavior. *Journal Health and Social Behavior 17*, December, 328-39

Knapp, David and Knapp, Deanne (1962). Decision making and self-medication: preliminary findings. *American Journal of Hosp. Pharm. 29*, December

Knapp, D.E., Baird, J.T. and Winters, W.J. (1976). How consumers view drugs. *The Apothecary 88*, 7-10, 38, August

Knoben, J.E. and Wertheimer, A. (1976). Physician prescribing patterns: therapeutic categories and age considerations. *Drug Intelligence and Clin. Pharm. 10*, 398, July

Kornetsky, C. (1976). *Pharmacology: Drugs Affecting Behavior*, New York, John Wiley and Sons

Korsch, B.M. and Negrete, V.F. (1972). Doctor-patient communication. *Scientific American, 227*, 66-72

Lasagna, L. and Epstein, L.C. (1969). Obtaining informed consent. *Arch. Intern. Med. 123*, June

Lasagna, L. and Joubert, P. (1975). Patient package inserts. I. nature, notions, and needs. *Clinical Pharmacology and Therapeutics 18*, 5, Part 1, November

—— (1975). Patient package inserts. II. toward a rational patient package insert. *Clinical Pharmacology and Therapeutics 18*, 6, December

Lasagna, L. (1969). Obtaining informed consent. *Arch. Intern. Med. 123*, June

Lasagna, L. and Stolley (1969). *Journal Chronic Dis. 22*, 395-405

Lawson, D.H. (1976). Drug prescribing in hospitals, an international comparison. *AJPH 66*, 7, July

Lennard, H.L. and Epstein, L.J. *et al.* (1971). *Mystification and Drug Misuse*, San Francisco, Jossey-Bass Inc

Ley, P. and Spelman, M.S. (1967). *Communicating with the Patient*, London, Staples Press

Ley, P. *et al.* (1976). Improving doctor-patient communication in general practice. *Journal of the Royal College of General Practitioners 26*, 720-4

Ley, P., Goldman, M., Bradshaw, P.W., Kincey, J.A. and Walker, C.M. (1972). Comprehensibility of some X-ray leaflets. *Journal of the Institute of Health Education 10*, 47-55

Ley, P. (1977). Psychological studies of doctor-patient communication. In *Contributions to Medical Psychology*, Rachman, S. (Ed.), Oxford, Pergamon Press, 9-42

Lilja, J. (1976). How physicians choose their drugs. *Soc. Science and Medicine 10*, 373-5

Lima, J. *et al.* (1976). Compliance with short term antimicrobial therapy: some techniques that help. *Pediatrics 57*, March, 383

Lovius, J., Lovius, B.B. and Ley, P. (1973). Comprehensibility of the literature given to patients at a dental hospital. *Journal of Public Health Dentistry 33*, 23-6

Madden, E. (1973). Evaluation of outpatient pharmacy patient counseling. *Journal of American Pharmaceutical Association NS 13*, 8, August

Malleson, A. (1973). *Need Your Doctor be so Useless?* London, George Allen and Unwin, Ltd

Matarazzo, J.D. and Saslow, G. (1960). Psychological and related characteristics of smokers and non-smokers. In *Psychology Bulletin 57*, 493-513

Mattar, M.E. *et al.* (1975). Pharmaceutic factors affecting pediatric compliance. *Pediatrics 55*(1), January, 101-8

Matthews, V.L. and Feather, J. (1976). Utilization of Health Services in Western Canada: Basic Canadian Data from WHO/International Collaborative Study of Medical Care Utilization. *CMA Journal 114*, February, 309

Mazzullo, J.M. (1976). Methods of improving patient compliance. *Drug Therapy 6*, March, 148

Mazzullo, J.M., Lasagna, L. and Griner, P.F. (1974). Variations in interpretations of prescription instructions: the need for improved prescribing habits. *JAMA 227*, 8, February

Mechanic, D. (1976). The growth of bureaucratic medicine: an inquiry into the dynamics of patient behavior and the organization of medical care, New York, John Wiley and Sons

McCree, C. *et al.* (1974). Psychiatrists response to sexual bias in pharmaceutical advertising. *American Journal of Psychiatry*

McIntire, M.S. *et al.* (1977). Safety packaging: what does the public think? *American Journal Public Health 67*, 69-171

McIntire, M.D., Angle, C.R. and Grush, M.I. (1976). How effective is safety packaging? *Clin. Toxicology 9*, 3, 419-25

McKenney, J. *et al.* (1973). The effect of clinical pharmacy services on patients with essential hypertension. *Circulation 47*, November, 1104

McKenney, J.M. and Harrison, W.L. (1976). Drug related hospital admissions. *American Journal Hospital Pharm. 33*(8), August, 792-5

McKeown, T. (1976). *The Role of Medicine: Dream, Mirage, or Nemesis?* London, Nuffield Provincial Hospitals Trust

Merrill, M.H. *et al.* (1958). Attitudes of Californians toward poliomyelitis vaccination. *American Journal Public Health 48*, 146-52

Milanski, R.J. *et al.* (1975). TV drug advertising and proprietary and illicit drug use among teenaged boys. *Public Opinion Quarterly 39*, Winter

Miller, R.R. (1979). Prescribing habits of physicians: a review of studies on prescribing drugs. Miller, R. (Ed.), Parts I-III *Drug Intelligence and Clinical Pharmacy 7*, Nov. 1973, Parts VII-VIII, *8*, Feb. 1974, 81-91

Morris, J.N. (1957). *Uses of Epidemiology*, Edinburgh and London, E. and S. Livingstone, Ltd

Moser, R.H. (1964). *Diseases of Medical Progress*, Springfield, Ill., C.C. Thomas

Muller, C. (1967). The study of prescribing as a technique of examining a medical care system. *AJPH 57* (12), 2117-25

National Council of Churches Drug Advertising Project (1973). Final report of Hearings on Drug Advertising, *2*, National Council of Churches of Christ, Washington, D.C., March

National Research Council, Division of Medical Sciences (1969). *Drug Efficacy Study*, Washington National Academy of Sciences

New York Times (1976). AMA Article, Department of Drugs, January 28

Nickerson, H. (1972). Patient education. *Health Education Monographs 31*, 95-97

Out-of-Pocket Cost and Acquisiton of Prescribed Medicines (1977). Data from the National Health Survey, 1973, US Department of Health, Education and Welfare, Public Health Service, Health Resources Administration, National Center for Health Statistics, Rockville, Md., June

Parish, P. (1974). The family doctor's role in psychotropic drug use. (1974). In Cooperstock, *Social Aspects of Medical Use in Psychotropic Drugs*, Addiction Research Foundation of Ontario

Peterson, B. *et al.* (1976). Television advertising and drug use. *AJPH 66*, (10)

Peterson, O.L. (1956). An analytical study of North Carolina general practice. *Journal Medical Ed. 31*, Pt. II, December

Pratt, L. (1976). *Family Structure and Effective Health Behavior: The Energized Family*, Boston, Houghton Mifflin

Pratt, L. *et al.* (1958). Physicians' views on medical information among patients in Gartley Jaco, E. *Patients, Physicians and Illness*, Illinois, Glencoe Free Press

Prutting, J. (1978). Autopsies – benefits for clinicians. *American Journal Clinical Pathology 69*, Suppl. 1, 223-5

Rabin, C. and Bush, D. (1974). The use of medicines. *Int. Journal Health Services 4*, 1, 61-87

Robinson, G. and Merav, A. (1976). Informed consent: recall by patients tested postoperatively. *Ann. Thorac. Surg. 22* (3), September, 209-12

Roper, B.W. (1973). Survey of public attitudes toward media. TV Information Office, *NAB* (745, 5th Ave., New York)

Rosser, W.W. (1975). A national self-evaluation programe for Canadian family doctors. (1975). *CMA Journal 112*, April 19

Rucker, T.D. (1976). Drug information for prescribers and dispensers: toward a model system. *Medical Care 13*, 2, February, 156-65

Ruskin, A. (1979). Survey of drug information needs and problems associated with communications directed to practising physicians. (1974). National Technical Information Services, Springfield, Va

Ryan, P.B. *et al.* (1975). Economic justification of pharmacist involvement in patient medication consultation. *American Journal Hospital Pharm. 32*(4), April, 389-92

Sackett, D.L. and Haynes, R.B. (Eds.) (1976). *Compliance with Therapeutic Regimens*, Baltimore, Johns Hopkins University Press

Salisbury, R. (1977). The pharmacist's duty to warn the patient of side effects of drugs. *Journal of the American Pharmaceutical Association NS 17*, (2) February

Scherz, R.G. (1974). Child proofing the medicine bottle. *Lancet 2*, 287

Schulz, P.E. and Perrier, C.V. (1976). Inadequacy of information about drugs. *Int. Journal Clinical Pharmacology 14*, (4), 255-8

Science News (1977). Female hormones and birth defects. *3*, January 22

Seidenberg, R. (1971). Drug advertising and perception of mental illness. *Mental Hygiene 55*, 21-31

Seltzer, C., Friedman, G. and Sieglaub, A.B. (1974). Smoking and drug consumption in white, black and oriental men and women. *American Journal Public Health 64*, 446-73

Sharpe, T. and Mikeal, R. (1974). Patient compliance with antibiotic regimens. *American Journal Hosp. Pharm. 31*, May, 479-84

Sheppard, C. *et al.* (1974). Comparative study of psychiatrists' treatment preferences: California and New York. *Comprehensive Psychiatry 15*, (3), 213

Shor, R.E. and Easton, R.D. (1975). Information processing analysis of the Chevreul Pendulum illusion. *Journal of Experimental Psychology: Human Perception and Performance 104*, (3), August, 231-6

Silverman, M. (1976). *The Drugging of the Americas*, Berkeley, University of California Press

Silverman, M. and Lee, P. (1974). *Pills, Profits and Politics*, Berkeley, US Press
Smith, M.C. (1976). How drug costs affect patient compliance. *Drug Therapy* 6, November, 87
—— (1977a). Appeals used in advertisements for psychotropic drugs: an exploratory study. *AJPH 67*, (2), February
—— (1977b). Drug product advertising and prescribing: a review of the evidence. *American Journal of Hospital Pharmacy 34*, 1208-24, November
Soueif, M.I. (1967). Hashish consumption in Egypt, with special reference to psychosocial problems. *Bulletin on Narcotics*, 19/2, 1-12
—— (1978). Personal Communication
Stimson, G.V. (1977). Do drug advertisements provide therapeutic information? *Journal of Medical Ethics 3*, 7-13
—— (1975c). Information contained in drug advertisements. *British Medical Journal 4*, November 29, 508-9
—— (1976a). The extent of advertising of pharmaceutical products. In *Prescribing in General Practice*, Parish, P.A., Stimson, G.V. and Mapes, R.E.A. (Eds.). *Journal of the Royal College of General Practitioners*, Supplement (1), 26, 69, 76
—— (1976b). The use of references in drug advertisements. In *Prescribing in General Practice*, Parish, P.A., Stimson, G.V. and Mapes, R.E. A. (Eds.). *Journal of the Royal College of General Practitioners*, Supplement (1), 26, 69, 76
—— (1975a). The message of psychotropic drug ads. *Media and Medicine*. Reprinted from *Journal of Communication*, Summer, *25* (3), 153-60
—— (1975b). Women in a doctored world. *New Society*, May 1, *32*, 265-7
Stokes, C.S. and Dudley, C. (1972). Family planning and conjugal roles. *Social Science and Medicine 6*, 157-61
Stolley, P.D. *et al.* (1972). The relationship between physician characteristics and prescribing appropriateness. *Medical Care 10*, 17-28
—— (1972). Drug prescribing and use in an American community. *Ann. Intern. Med. 76*, 1, 537
Task Force of Prescription Drugs, The Drug Users (1968). Washington, US Government Printing Office
US Department of Health, Education and Welfare (1969). *The Task Force on Prescription Drugs: The Users*, US Government Printing Office, 36
Wadsworth, M.E.J. (1974). Health and sickness: the choice of treatment. *Journal Psychosom. Research 18*, (4), August, 271
Wadsworth, M.E.J. *et al.* (1971). *Health and Sickness, The Choice of Treatment*, London, Tavistock Publications
Wardell, W.M. (1973). Introduction of new therapeutic drugs in the United States and Great Britain: an international comparison. *Clin. Pharmacol. Therap. 14*, 773
White, K.L. *et al.* (1961). The ecology of medical care. *New England Journal of Medicine 265*, 885
Wickware, D.S. (1977). What practitioners think about PPIs. *Patient Care*, February 1
Woodcock, J. (1976). Speaking of education: approaches. Quoted in Blum, R., Blum, E., and Garfield, E. *Drug Education: Results and Recommendations*, Lexington, Mass., D.C. Heath and Company
Zborowski, M. (1952). Cultural components in response to pain. *Social Issues 8*, 16-30
Zola, I.K. (1972). Studying the decision to see a doctor: review, critique, corrective, *Adv. in Psychosom. Med. 8*, 216-36
—— (1973). Pathways to the doctor – from person to patient. *Soc. Sci. and Med. 7*

7 ECONOMIC CONSIDERATIONS IN THE PROVISION AND USE OF MEDICINES[1]

Sanjaya Lall

7.1 Introduction

This chapter deals with a narrower field than its title suggests. It does not go into the entire range of issues concerning the economics of the pharmaceutical industry.[2] This would be an enormous task, and would not in any case be particularly relevant to the objectives of this book. It concentrates on the provision of medicines to the less-developed countries (LDCs), and tries to highlight the deficiencies in the existing market system by which this provision is made. As the bulk of medicines in less-developed countries is provided by large, transnational companies (TNCs) originating in the advanced industrial nations, we devote some attention to market structure in developed countries, but most of our attention is given to the problems that their operations raise in the Third World.

The focus of this chapter is thus the provision of drugs to the LDCs by multinational companies. It is argued that the oligopolistic structure of the industry (with a relatively few large companies dominating international production, trade and innovation) lends considerable market power to the large firms, and that the exercise of this market power entails a number of costs — economic and social — for the LDCs which rely on this system of drug delivery.

In Section 7.2 we describe the structure of the industry, and the growth of concentration over time. In Section 7.3 we discuss some indications of the monopolistic or market power, which suggest that the leading firms do possess competitive advantages over small ones, and so are able to earn higher profits, charge higher prices and exercise greater influence on the prescribers. In Section 7.4 the implications of this system are drawn for the LDCs. Section 7.5 closes with some policy recommendations.

7.2 Concentration in the Pharmaceutical Industry

We consider concentration in two forms: geographical and
structural. The former serves to show how drug production is
distributed between the developed and less-developed worlds. The
latter provides a preliminary indication of the dominance of the
MNCs in international drug production.

As far as *geographical* concentration is concerned, data are not
uniformly available for all countries. For socialist countries, it is
difficult to convert production figures meaningfully from local
currencies to dollar values; for a number of LDCs, figures are not
available or not very reliable. However, in an earlier publication
(Lall, 1978a), I had made certain estimates for production and
consumption of drugs in 1973 in 48 'market economy' (i.e. non-
socialist, but including Yugoslavia) countries. These figures,
while subject to many weaknesses, do give a fairly accurate picture
of the broad orders of magnitude, and are shown in Table 7.1
below.

The developed countries accounted, in 1973, for nearly 85
per cent of world production. The LDCs, while containing some
three-quarters of the world's population, accounted for 10 per cent
of production and 13 per cent of consumption. More recent figures
show that the industry, while growing rapidly everywhere, is expanding
faster in the LDCs than in the developed countries. However, the
overwhelming dominance of the developed economies is likely to
continue for the foreseeable future.

Table 7.1: Estimated Production and Consumption of Pharmaceuticals,
1973 ($ million)

Area	Number of Countries	Production Value	%	Consumption[a] Value	%
Developed (non-socialist)	17	24,919	84.4	23,372	80.8
South European[b]	4	1,534	5.2	1,789	6.2
Less-deveoped (non-socialist)[c]	27	3,113	10.4	3,767	13.0
Total	48	29,556	100.0	28.937	100.0

Source: S. Lall, (1978). *The Growth of the Pharmaceutical Industry in
Developing Countries*, Vienna, UNIDO.
Notes: [a] Defined as production plus imports minus exports. [b] Spain, Portugal,
Greece and Turkey. [c] Including Yugoslavia.

Within the developed world, the six leading producers (France, Germany, Italy, Japan, UK and US) account for nearly 75 per cent of world output. In this group, Japan, Germany and Italy are growing faster than others (production figures for Switzerland are not available), while the US was slowly losing its share of the world market. As far as exports are concerned, the seven leading exporters (excluding Japan from the above but including Switzerland and the Netherlands) accounted for nearly 80 per cent of the non-socialist world's exports.

Within the less-developed world, Brazil, India, Mexico, Argentina and Egypt are leading producers (we exclude Spain and Yugoslavia from this group). These are the countries which have managed to achieve a considerable degree of backward integration in drug manufacture. India, in particular, is able to make the greater part of its needs entirely within the country.

The geographical pattern of innovation is even more concentrated than that of production. Only a handful of countries, with the US far ahead of others (mainly UK, West Germany, France, Switzerland), have contributed significantly to the discovery of new medicines in the last 40 years.[3] While the pace of innovation has slowed down significantly in the last decade, and the decline has been most marked in the US, the overall pattern of innovation as between developed and less-developed countries has not changed. The developed countries still contribute, and will continue to contribute, almost all important discoveries in the medical field, despite the rapidly escalating costs of conducting research and development (R and D) the difficulties of introducing new drugs, and the efforts of LDCs to attract TNCs' research investments.

As far as *structural* concentration is concerned, some estimates for worldwide production by the leading TNCs are shown in Table 7.2 below. Comparing 1970 with 1974, it appears that there has been a slight increase in the share of the large companies at all levels of measurement. By 1974, the top 30 firms accounted for over half of the non-socialist world's production of drugs. At a rough guess, the top 100 firms accounted for about 70 per cent, and several thousand smaller firms in developed and less developed countries accounted for the remainder.

A first glance at these overall figures suggests that the level of concentration here is not high relative to other industries where multinationals are active (e.g. automobiles, computers and electricals). Concentration levels within particular countries are similarly low by comparison: the leading firm in each developed country accounts

Table 7.2: Worldwide Concentration of Pharmaceutical Sales, 1970 and 1974, ($ million)

	1970		1974	
	Sales	%	Sales	%
Total Market Economy Sales	18,633	100.0	34,001	100.0
Sales of 10 leading firms	4,987	26.7	9,498	27.9
Sales of 20 leading firms	7,748	41.5	14,561	42.8
Sales of 30 leading firms	9,429	49.6	17,682	52.0

Source: Lall (1978a).

for under 10 per cent of the total drug market. In 1973, the leading 4 firms in the US accounted for 28 per cent, and in the UK 29 per cent, of the total market; the leading 20 firms accounted for 76 per cent and 75 per cent respectively.[4] The tendency over time has been for concentration to decrease in the UK and for a slight decrease followed by a slight increase in the US. In general terms, however, there are few signs that the tendency to increasing monopolisation that marks most 'modern' (i.e. non-traditional) manufacturing industries is manifested in the pharmaceutical sector.

The evolution of market structures is the outcome of several, often conflicting, forces. In the pharmaceutical industry, the main determinant of high concentration levels in sectors like steel or automobiles – economies of scale in production – is absent at the level of formulation. There *are* scale economies further back in the production chain (especially production of fine chemicals), but this need not cause concentration at the level of furnished drug production. A large number of formulators can (and do) produce the final drug competitively by buying the intermediate chemical from a few firms. Given this, the observed changes in structure (the determinants of concentrations as such are discussed in the next section) must be traced to other factors.

These factors are essentially related to the innovative process (and to its concomitant, the emergence of competition for older drugs) within each pharmaceutical submarket.[5] In submarkets where new drug introductions are relatively rapid, the level of concentration tends to increase, for two reasons: the legal quasi-monopoly granted by the patent system, and the increasing costs of innovation and new drug introduction. In submarkets where, on the other hand, there is a prevalence of older drugs, for which patents have expired or imitations have appeared, we observe greater competition and lower levels of concentration.[6] The overall structure thus reflects the balance between the 'innovative' and 'established' drug markets.

As far as the 'innovative' markets are concerned, the literature has remarked on the phenomenon of a marked slow-down in the introduction of new drugs. This has been a worldwide tendency, but concern has been expressed in the US that the slow-down is greater than in other developed countries.[7] Several reasons have been advanced for this trend: a 'plateau' in scientific possibilities for new discoveries; higher R and D costs; official stringency in new drug introduction, adding considerably to the time and money required for establishing the safety of new medicines; price controls and declining profits. This is a controversial topic in which the debate (between the industry and government) usually revolves around the pros and cons of official regulation, and we shall not enter into it here, It should suffice to note that the level of concentration *in innovation* has risen markedly in recent years, and may be expected to continue increasing in the future.

The levels of concentration found within individual therapeutic categories (which are separate markets in the economic sense) is, as may be expected, much higher than for the pharmaceutical market as a whole.[8] In general, they approach levels found in other modern manufacturing industries (70-80 per cent of the market being held by the leading four firms), though there is some variation around this range. The picture is fairly dynamic over time. Several submarkets in the UK, for instance, show declines in concentration levels, and about the same number show increases (see Table 7.3). Furthermore, the identity of the market leaders changes frequently, showing intense rivalry among the larger firms within the therapeutic categories in which they specialise.

The fact that such active oligopolistic competition exists among the large drug companies is sometimes taken by industry protagonists to show that there is *no* market power in the industry (not, at least, over the long term), and to support their case for de-control of the market. (We return to this below.) It is maintained here, however, that active competition can co-exist among market leaders with a considerable degree of market power enjoyed by these leaders *as a group* (in relation to smaller rivals). The methods by which this market power is acquired lead, moreover, to serious social costs, especially in LDCs. At the same time, they yield some important

Table 7.3: Concentration of 30 Leading Therapeutic Categories in the UK 1964 and 1973 (Percentages)

Rank* Therapeutic class		Share of Leading Firm		Share of Four Leading Companies	
		1964	1973	1964	1973
1	Broad-spectrum antibiotics	39%	42%	99%	80%
2	Systemic anti-inflammatories	80	40	98	88
3	Bronchodilators	32	42	63	82
4	Other hypertensives	62	67	98	91
5	Diuretics	51	40	75	80
6	Non-narcotic analgesics	29	30	68	70
7	Anti-depressants	39	23	89	61
8	Tranquillisers	45	53	88	83
9	Anti-angina	34	63	74	93
10	Plain skin hormones	44	53	88	87
11	Cough remedies	41	42	66	69
12	Plain antacids	31	34	68	65
13	Contraceptives	23	33	65	82
14	Non-barbiturates	34	72	86	95
15	Peripheral vasodilators	42	31	75	80
16	Systemic antibiotics	41	32	86	90
17	Haematinics	26	31	51	81
18	Anti-nauseants	55	34	91	82
19	Penicillin	26	26	69	74
20	Anti-infective skin hormones	17	23	64	59
21	Anti-obesity preparations	23	60	77	94
22	Laxatives	31	30	72	70
23	ACTH-systemic hormones	27	20	76	60
24	Oral anti-diabetic	57	44	99	93
25	Parkinson anticonvulsants	41	40	87	89
26	Antispasmodics	35	16	73	54
27	Systemic antihistamines	30	24	83	66
28	TB preparations	40	34	86	95
29	Oral cold preparations	44	53	92	90
30	Other vitamins	60	40	93	92

*Ranked according to 1973 sales volume.
Source: Slatter (1977), 49.

benefits, especially in terms of providing major innovations. We turn now to these considerations.

7.3 Indicators and Sources of Market Power

The level of concentration in an industry is the most commonly used indicator of the existence of market power, but it is only one of several others. According to this indicator, the drug industry seems to be possessed of considerable market power at the therapeutic group level, though evidence of competition between the market leaders may be used to persuade us that this is not so. Two further tasks await us: to see whether other indicators of market power support the hypothesis that, despite oligopolistic rivalry, the market leaders retain considerable market power; and, if so, what consequence the process of oligopolistic rivalry and competitive acquisition of market power has for social welfare. The first of these is dealt with in this section, the second in the next.

In an earlier paper (1975), I had discussed three other indicators of market power in the pharmaceutical industry. Let us remark on them briefly:

Price Discrepancies. The drug industry exhibits substantial price differences (1) between regions, buyers and countries (indicating the power to discriminate between markets, the classic sign of market power), and (2) between identical products sold under brand names by large firms and those sold under generic names by small ones.

(1) While data on price discrimination by drug firms are, in the nature of the matter, difficult to find, the few figures that exist show significant differences, especially between countries, that cannot be explained simply by reference to exchange rate changes, regulations, transport cost, and the like.[9] Roche's 'Librium' and 'Valium', for instance, were priced from 700 per cent and 1100 per cent higher in the US than in the UK in 1975; other examples are mentioned in my (1975) study.

(2) Price differences between identical branded and generic products in the pharmaceutical industry are better known and recorded, especially in the United States. Evidence before the US Senate hearings since the early 1960s has in fact covered innumerable such cases, and it would hardly be useful to give further figures if it were not for recent attempts by the industry's defenders to establish that price competition was flourishing and effective in pharmaceutical markets.[10] Using data on price declines of drugs, especially of antibiotics (which have experienced the most dramatic price reductions of any class of drugs), they have argued that drug firms could not be accused of possessing excessive market power when competition clearly affected their pricing policies.

This is an important argument which, if valid, would have serious implications for the case advanced in this paper and for the whole gamut of regulatory policies set up by various governments to control pharmaceutical prices. The industry's case is, however, unfounded and the argument of its defenders misleading and misdirected. It is misdirected because critics have not claimed that large drug companies were absolute monopolists which could ignore all actual and potential competition: clearly, they are oligopolists who must take each other's reactions into account in all matters, including pricing. It is misleading because it uses evidence on oligopolistic rivalry (between the large firms) to deduce that competition is fully effective. In fact, since competition in the drug industry is largely confined to the dominant firms,[11] such evidence does not prove or disprove that large firms as such continue to exercise substantial market power *vis à vis* their small rivals. We have to look at prices in multi-source markets, where large and small suppliers co-exist, to see whether prices are in fact significantly different, and whether large firms are able to maintain dominant market shares despite higher prices.

A recent study of Brooke (1975) provides just such evidence on antibiotic markets in the US. Some of Brooke's main findings are

Table 7.4: Price Differentials[a] in US Antibiotics Markets Between Large and Small Firms (1972) (US dollars)

Drug	Dominant Supplier		Largest Five Suppliers		Lowest Available Price
	Price	Market Share (%)	Average Price	Market Share (%)	
1. Erythromycin	12.96	46	9.91	80	5.70
2. Potassium Penicillin	8.36	78[c]	5.40[e]	over 90[e]	1.20
3. Penicillin VK	8.32	52	7.21	88	1.85
4. Oxytetracycline	18.43	96	–	–	1.90
5. Tetracycline	22.70	35	22.52	86	4.12
6. Ampicillin	13.81	24	10.62	72	4.40
7. Chloramphenicol	23.71	99	–	–	app. 7.90
8. Sulfisoxazole	22.50	n.a.[d]	n.a.	n.a.	8.90

Source: Lall (1978 b) Appendix 1, calculated from Brooke's (1975) various tables.
Notes:
    a. 'Average transaction price' for the main dosage form of the drug.
    b. Market shares calculated for the main dosage form of the drug.
    c. Market share for total potassium penicillin market.
    d. Exact market share not available, but price quoted is for firm known to be dominant.
    e. Two firms only.

displayed in Table 7.4, and they show clearly that 'competition' in pharmaceutical markets does not eliminate great market power in the hands of large firms. Such firms are able to retain large shares of the market despite charging prices which are often several times higher than prices charged for identical products by smaller firms. Since these products are all 'multi-source' and not protected by patents the reason for price differentials lies (as argued below) in brand preference created by promotion.

The Earning of Exceptionally High Profits. These are earned by the industry as a whole, and, within it, by the dominant firms, over long periods of time. Despite recent declines in profitability caused by the recession, pharmaceuticals remain one of the two or three most profitable sectors in manufacturing industry, in developed as well as less-developed countries. There are some problems about determining the economically correct rate of profit in this industry – the treatment of R and D expenses,[12] the allowance for risk, the correct calculation of the capital base, and, most important, the determination of correct transfer prices on intra-firm transactions. The industry is well known for the latitude with which its transfer prices are assigned, a result of the highly firm-specific nature of the intermediates traded between different units of given TNCs. Studies in LDCs and developed countries alike reveal that TNCs use these prices to shift profits out of areas where it is costly or risky to declare high profits.[13] In some cases the device is used to push up costs, and so prices negotiated with authorities: a recent example for Europe is given by M. Dondelinger, a Belgian member of the European Parliament, according to whom 'Metoclopramide is manufactured in Caen, France, by Laboratoire Delaire at a price of Fr. 100 per kilo in bulk.' The drug then 'passes from subsidiary to subsidiary through Belgium and ends up in Switzerland, near Zurich, under the label of the Zofingen company.' The European MP alleges that Zofingen 'then resells it officially in foreign economy "to Delagrage" who pays Fr. 4,000 a kilo, packages it and distributes it to chemists where it is sold to the public at the price approved by the Ministry of Health of Fr. 8,000 per kilo.'[14]

If these problems were all taken into account the declared rate of profit in many countries – high as it is – would probably be higher still. In Sri Lanka, for instance, some TNC subsidiaries engaged in local manufacture were found to be importing pharmaceutical chemicals from their principals at prices 3-4 times higher than charged by *other TNCs*: the drugs involved were fairly old and out of patent, so that 'contribution to R and D' (the standard reason advanced for changing high transfer prices) could hardly be used to justify the practice.[15]

The profit performance of the industry, and especially of the dominant firms, thus confirms the existence of entry barriers suggested by other indicators.

Product Differentiation and High Levels of Promotional Expenditures. These can serve both as an indicator as well as a cause of market power. In this industry, despite the 'scientific' nature of its users and products, both these indicators suggest very intense efforts to create market power. Some 700-1,000 drugs are sold under several thousand brand names in almost every country, and the average level of promotional expenditure is one of the highest of all manufacturing industries. Table 7.5 sets out some recent data on this. It should be noted that these average promotional expenses conceal considerable variation. On most newly launched or heavily marketed products the expense is much higher; in some cases, particularly if the product fails to capture a large section of the market, promotion expenses may *exceed* the total value of sales.[16]

The industry is notorious for its use of high-pressure sales techniques, and it is being forced in every advanced country to reduce its spending on promotion, to control the content of its advertising and to offer less obvious benefits to doctors who prescribe its products. In less-developed countries the controls are less strict, and there is reason to believe that the hold of promotion over doctors is stronger.[17]

All indicators, then, support the case that the dominant firms exercise considerable market power in the drug industry. This is not

Table 7.5: Promotional Expenditure and Number of Drug Specialities in Selected Countries

Country	Promotional Expenditures as % of Sales	Approximate No. of Product Specialities
US	22	35,000 or more
UK	15	10,000
W. Germany	22	12,000-15,000
Italy	22	15,600
Sweden	18	1,650
France	17	6,500
India	18	15,000

Sources: Slatter (1977), Tables 5.2 and 6.2, and Lall (1975).

to assert that this power is stable. As we have noted, the existence of intense oligopolistic competition leads to frequent changes in market leadership within particular therapeutic categories, depending on the ability of the large firms to innovate and market new products. Furthermore, economic stringency and a growing realisation of the problems raised by the strategies of large firms (which we discuss below) have led various governments to become increasingly strict about the introduction of 'new' drugs which offer little therapeutic benefit, to cut down on promotional excesses and to control prices directly. This has caused some containment of the market power of the large firms (though not necessarily a reduction in concentration levels), a tendency which may be strengthened by the innovational slowing down in the industry. This slowing down has meant that in many important therapeutic groups (led by antibiotics) leading products are coming to the end of patent protection and so facing competition from the branded products of large rivals and generic products of small rivals.

While the proportion of generic prescriptions written is still small (about 12 per cent in the US,[18] and much less in Continental Europe), the importance of multi-source markets is bound to increase over the next few years, and generic prescribing is also likely to grow under official urging. It is not certain, however, that this will necessarily lead to a weakening in the competitive position and market shares of the large drug companies. As we saw earlier, their branded products continue to dominate markets and fetch higher prices even when several smaller competitors exist. The latest evidence suggests that, by aggressively attacking generic markets and launching their own generic products as they are forced into them, 'the major companies look set to retain their dominant positions'.[19] The loss of one source of market power (technology) has naturally led the firms to rely more on the other (marketing); the final result does not seem to be very different, and dominant firms remain dominant.

Let us now consider briefly the *sources* of market power. The two main supports of market power in pharmaceuticals are (1) technology and (2) marketing.

Technology. The ability to produce new drugs — whether they are major advances, minor improvements or simply imitations or new combinations — are the lifeblood of growth in the industry. The institution of the patent system is of prime significance here. This system provides a legal monopoly to innovators for 17-20 years in

most countries,[20] though its effective life is less because of the time
lag between registering a patent and bringing a product on the market.
Unlike other industries where the growing importance of unpatented
know-how has reduced the significance of patents in protecting
innovation, the pharmaceutical sector remains crucially dependent on
patents to protect earnings on new products. The role of patents in
LDCs, however, seems to be mainly to protect the export markets
of TNCs; a tiny fraction, under 5 per cent of the total patents taken
out by innovators, are actually used for production there. While patents
are in force, the host country is obliged to import the products at the
prices charged by the TNCs, regardless of the availability of similar
products at much lower prices from imitating firms.

As far as new products are concerned, the tendency to increased
concentration in R and D, coupled with the institutional framework
of patents, provides a growing source of market power. As far as
existing products are concerned, the innovational structure of the
industry provides a strong incentive to produce imitative or slightly
modified drugs which can (a) extend the effective life of the original
patent (for the innovator), or (b) get around the original patent (for
an imitator), or (c) provide a medicine (say, a new 'combination' of
existing drugs) which can be marketed as a new product, or (d) provide
a product which can be sold as appropriate to slightly different
indications. There is controversy over how much this sort of product
competition adds to the market power and earnings of drug companies:
what is clear is that, in the absence of strong regulation by the government, the great bulk of 'new' drugs sold are of an imitative or trivial
nature (see also Chapter 3).

Take the US case. Table 7.6 gives the most recent figures on the
FDA's classification of 1,935 drugs up to April 1977. The products
covered are in the 'Investigational New Drug' (IND) phase. Practically
all of them are introduced by the large firms. The tests of the FDA
show that only 3.3 per cent of total new drugs constitute important
therapeutic gains, and less than 20 per cent constitute even modest
gains. The vast majority of IND registrations are trivial, and 45 per
cent of the total are new formulations, combinations or imitations
(items 3, 4 and 5) under category C, derived from R and D directed
at what is commonly known as 'molecule manipulation'. Although
some results of such R and D do lead to therapeutic gains, it appears
that this is more a by-product of marketing-orientated research than
the main product of genuinely innovational research. Cox, Millane and
Styles (1975) describe the alternative research policies pharmaceutical

Table 7.6: US Classification of New IND Drugs by Therapeutic Value by FDA (as of April, 1977)

Type of Drug Introduction	A Important Therapeutic Gain		B Modest Gain		C Little or No Gain		Dᵃ Other		Totalᵇ	
	No.	%	No.	%	No.	%	No.	%	No.	%
(1) New molecular entity	50	78.1	167	55.8	538	35.0	20	57.1	775	40.0
%	6.4		21.5		69.4		2.5		100.0	
(2) New salt, ester or derivative	2	3.1	19	6.3	137	8.9	1	2.8	159	8.2
%	1.2		11.9		86.1		0.6		100.0	
(3) New combination or formulation	5	7.8	69	23.0	242	15.7	3	8.5	319	16.4
%	1.5		21.6		75.8		0.9		100.0	
(4) Already marketed drug	2	3.1	25	8.3	445	28.9	3	8.5	475	24.5
%	0.4		5.2		93.6		0.6		100.0	
(5) Already marketed by same firm	5	7.8	19	6.3	175	11.3	8	22.8	207	10.6
%	2.4		9.1		84.5		3.8		100.0	
(6) Totalᵇ	64	100.0	299	100.0	1,537	100.0	35	100.0	1,935	100.0
%	3.3		15.5		79.4		1.8		100.0	

Source: Scrip, 24th September, 1977, 13

Notes: ᵃ Includes 'special situation' drugs which offer decreased safety or effectiveness but have some compensating virtue, and drugs under review for being 'less than effective'. ᵇ Percentages may not sum up to 100 because of rounding.

companies may adopt and illustrate the crucial role of marketing-based research in providing a continuous stream of 'new' products.

One increasingly important aspect of drug innovation, stressed heavily by the drug companies themselves (Teeling-Smith, 1979), is that of the slow-down in innovation. This has, as noted above, several causes. If it continues, it will have important long-term consequences for the structure and functioning of the industry as we now know it, with fewer new medicines, greater competition for existing products and a rise in generic prescribing. We cannot, unfortunately, go more deeply into these fascinating questions here.

The Role of Marketing in Creating and Maintaining Positions of Market Power. This is as important as that of innovation. It is a commonly noted feature of consumer-product oligopolies that competition usually concentrates on product differentiation and new product introduction rather than on price rivalry. This tendency is strengthened in the pharmaceutical industry because the complete separation of identity between the buyer (the patient or whatever agency pays for the patient) and the decision-maker (the doctor) eliminates any direct pressure on the latter to 'economise' in the normal sense of the word.

In this situation it is only to be expected that manufacturers will aim to continually introduce 'new' products on the market with a barrage of high-powered promotion, the success of which depends on impressing on the doctor the virtues (in terms of their therapeutic superiority or better quality) of particular brand names. The instances in which lower price is stressed as a major selling-point are conspicuous by their rarity.[21] It is true that major therapeutic breakthroughs can be priced higher than minor ones, and that purely imitative drugs tend to be comparable in price to, or somewhat cheaper than, the originals (and so bring down the prices of leading drugs over time), but all drugs which can be promoted effectively can command a premium in price over unadvertised generics, and the effectiveness in selling a drug as 'new' does not always depend on its therapeutic novelty.

There is an intimate and vital link between the innovational and marketing functions of the large drug companies. Innovation requires a powerful promotional system to achieve commercial success; and an extensive marketing network requires a constant stream of 'new' products to feed it. When combined with a situation where there are few sources of objective information on drug efficacy, price and comparability available to the doctor, and those that are do not match the lavishness or effectiveness of drug company advertising, we have a market where true innovation is liberally mixed with imitation or molecule manipulation, where information on therapy is submerged in powerful promotion, and competition is subverted by brand preference.

While the more advanced countries are instituting measures to check on the effectiveness of drugs, to (as in France) regulate the prices of 'me-too' as opposed to genuinely new drugs, to control the expenditure on and content of advertising, and to provide some 'counter-promotion' to drug company marketing, the LDCs are generally far behind in such reform. Many of them are even uncon-scious of the problems raised by the normal mode of oligopolistic competition in the drug industry, and those that are face immense political and social difficulties in launching major reforms.[22]

7.4 Consequences of Market Power

It cannot be doubted that drug TNCs have made major contributions to the discovery of new drugs, to their worldwide production and distribution, and to the knowledge of new therapies on the part of the medical profession. In fact, given private enterprise in the industry and the course of scientific progress in chemotherapy, it is unlikely that any other system of R and D, production and marketing could have yielded better results.

This being said, however, it must be admitted that the industry's mode of operations has entailed substantial direct and indirect costs in most host countries, especially the poor ones, costs which can be reduced by appropriate regulatory action. To mention them briefly:

Direct Costs. The direct costs of the industry may be defined as those which show up in the prices charged by TNCs. They are 'costs' to host countries in the sense that an alternative means of drug provision — and a range of alternatives is conceivable, as discussed in the section on policy — could supply the same effective medication at lower prices. There are three elements which constitute direct costs in this sense:

(1) Profits: while a normal rate of profit, taking into account the riskiness of investment (especially in R and D), is a necessary cost of production, it can be plausibly argued that in the pharmaceutical industry the actual profitability of the dominant firms is too high. As far as new drugs are concerned, the period of patent protection,

and the hold established by successful brand promotion, enables firms to earn returns which are not justified by the actual riskiness of the investment. The market power built up for new drugs persists even when competition appears (though it declines with the entry of large rivals), and permits profits to be earned by dominant firms that are higher than a truly competitive rate. The contribution of marketing-based entry barriers to profits is so apparent that it is difficult to accept the industry's claim that all higher-than-normal profits are due solely to the riskiness of R and D.

As far as LDCs are concerned, this cost is compounded by two factors. First, where transfer pricing is used to remit profit clandestinely, the host governments (and local shareholders, where relevant) do not even collect their legitimate share of the profits earned in the host economy. Second, where innovations are developed primarily for developed markets, and poor countries are made to contribute at the same rate as rich ones, it can be argued that the profit earned in LDCs is pure 'rent' which does not contribute to investment in R and D. In other words, even if LDCs paid no contribution to R and D on 'rich man's drugs', the expenditure on their innovation would continue unaffected: there is then no *economic* reason why they should make such contributions.

(2) Misdirected R and D: the prices charged for pharmaceutical products reflect not only the costs of genuine innovation but also the portion of R and D spent on trivial or imitative innovation. While Table 7.6 above showed that some such R and D has social benefits, most of it can probably be eliminated with little harm, indeed with considerable saving in scarce technical resources.

(3) Promotional expenditure: if the same information on drug therapy as provided by the enormous expenditures of drug firms could be effectively imparted at lower cost — and recent cuts imposed by various governments indicate that this is possible — then all the extra over that minimum is socially wasteful. It contributes to the market power of the firms concerned, but not to good therapy, and certainly not to the ability of the poor to buy medicines. If the information function were centralised, it is likely that the cost would be even further reduced, and that the present alternative system would show correspondingly higher social waste.

Indirect Costs. These costs do not show up in the high prices charged for drugs, but they are real none-the-less, especially in poor countries. To mention them very briefly:

(1) Overprescribing and misprescribing of drugs, leading to financial waste, unnecessary adverse reactions and building of resistance to drugs (one estimate for the US puts deaths caused by misprescribing at 30,000 per year), and the creation of drug dependence: all caused to some extent by the powerful promotional mechanisms used by the TNCs.

(2) Suppression of competition by small firms (of special significance to local competitors in developing countries) by the implicit denigration of the products of such firms in drug advertising by the multinationals, and by monopolistic practices in providing (or withholding) the essential 'active ingredients' required for drug formulation.[23] The licensing of drug technology is frequently hemmed in by a variety of restrictive business practices.

(3) Prescribing of the latest drugs which, by the income and health requirements of poor countries, are 'overeffective', in that the same medication, though perhaps with a higher incidence of adverse effects, could be provided by older and far cheaper drugs. The present system of drug provision renders a rational trade-off between cost and efficacy extremely difficult.

(4) Prescribing of a number of drugs (and their direct sale to consumers) which are ineffective, and do not do what is claimed for them.[24]

(5) Stultification of local R and D by creating total dependence on imported technology. Where the local government does undertake research (as in India), it has shown some success, proving that very large and sophisticated laboratories concentrated in developed countries are not essential for conducting worthwhile research. The most important advances have been made in improving and adapting processes; the R and D contribution of developing countries is negligible as far as important new products are concerned. However, there is a growing risk that research conducted locally within the existing structure will be picked up by the multinationals and commercialised by their parents.

(6) Selling without adequate warnings. The laxity of official control in developing areas often leads to drugs being sold without the warnings which are required in developed countries. Ledogar (1975) and Silverman (1976) provide a compendium of such cases for

Latin America; similar evidence could undoubtedly be collected in other LDCs.

(7) Clinical testing in developing countries when such testing has been strictly controlled in developed ones. The population of the former obviously bears the risk of proving the marketability of a drug by a foreign multinational.

The combined effect of these factors on developing countries is that drugs are too expensive, too 'modern', often overused by those who can afford them, and extremely *unequally distributed*. Only a small proportion of the population can afford to buy the drugs provided by the multinationals (80 per cent of the Indian population does not have access to drugs), and even they often mis-spend in relation to the benefits provided. Cheap and effective drugs are not provided to meet the real medical needs of the rest because this is not where the profits of the multinationals are made.

These 'costs' are, furthermore, not just that the present system happens to provide inappropriate and costly drugs to an élite, but also that, in the absence of an alternative system of drug production, innovation and marketing, it becomes impossible for developing countries to provide essential medicines to the majority of their populations. The existing system is, in other words, so pervasive and powerful that, *without major reform, it prevents the use of any easy alternative method of getting cheap and adequate supplies of essential drugs by poorer countries*. This is so partly because there are strong vested interests in these countries (including the medical profession) which support a continuing dependence on the drug multinationals, partly because there is strong faith in their branded products (in turn, partly because quality control of local firms may be inadequate), partly because of the technological backwardness of the chemical industries in developing countries (strengthened by the attitudes engendered by 'dependence'), and partly because of the weaknesses of their administrative structures.

7.5 Policy Options

The need for a reform of the system of pharmaceutical delivery to the poor of the world is now widely accepted by most LDCs, international agencies and (implicitly) by several TNCs themselves.[25] In fact, the reforms under discussion are essentially a combination of the various measures already taken by the developed countries to control the drug industry: [26] e.g. the FDA's attempts to introduce generic competition and check drug effectiveness; the UK attempt to restrain profitability; the French measures to check prices directly and to create a two-tier price structure for new and old drugs; the Swedish method of strictly controlling new drug registration; the German and French attempts to limit promotion; etc.

It has been argued above that minor reforms are likely to be ineffective in LDCs: the main reason for this is their urgent need for cheap, effective medication for the majority of their populations who cannot afford the vast array of expensive, modern drugs. This calls for a concentration of resources on meeting the most common ailments: on compiling what has become known as a 'basic' or 'essential' drug list.[27] While the drug industry is opposed to such a list (which would greatly reduce the scope for product differentiation, promotion and minor innovation) such strategy seems eminently sensible to meet the special conditions prevailing in LDCs.

The WHO Expert Committee on the Selection of Essential Drugs has drawn up an illustrative list of essential drugs, and the organisation has come out officially strongly in favour of such lists. This committee concluded in its final report that 'in the light of present scientific knowledge, a sample of about *200 essential drugs* (active substances) is indispensable for the health care of the vast majority of the world's population . . . For the optimum use of limited financial resources, the available drugs must be restricted to those proven to be thera-peutically effective, to have acceptable safety and to satisfy the health needs of the population'. It is recognised that 'a limited list may not provide for the needs of every person, but certainly should for the vast majority; whether or not drugs or pharmaceutical products outside the list are available in the private sector should be a local decision'.[28] The need to adapt the list to differing local conditions and to update it periodically is also stressed.

The drawing up of some priority list is only the first step in pharmaceutical reform. The next logical step would be to rationalise the whole list of drugs available in a country. This 'rationalised list' would contain some 600-800 drugs, including those on the 'essential' drug list, and would provide sufficient medication for secondary and tertiary health care (primary health care being met by essential drugs). The main aim of such rationalisation would be (1) to promote prescribing by generic and not brand names, (2) to cut out imitative products which add nothing to therapy, (3) to eliminate combination products which are therapeutically undesirable or which are ineffective, (4) to eliminate drugs with unacceptably high toxicity, and (5) to reduce the commercial pressures on the part of manufacturers to produce trivial 'new' drugs and to promote brand names.[29] While rationalisation is of greatest value in LDCs where economic pressures call for urgent economy and where official controls in brand-name promotion are slack, clearly a similar policy (along the lines of Sweden, which has a far smaller number of drugs on the market than, say, the US or Germany) in advanced countries would also have medical and economic benefits.

Whatever sort of essential or rationalised list a government adopts, there are likely to be severe problems in implementing it: quality and 'bioavailability' problems; resistance by the medical profession; pressures by the large drug companies; and hostility from the élite groups of consumers who are used to the whole array of expensive branded drugs. Thus, progress has to be very slow and careful. The government has to ensure that the drugs it obtains are of satisfactory quality and biologically equivalent with the branded drugs of the TNCs; both raise technical and administrative problems of great magnitude, and for a number of drugs bioequivalence of generic and branded products has not yet been established. It has to mount an education campaign aimed at the medical profession to raise their consciousness on generic prescribing, economising and the availability of good quality drugs from small generic producers. A sudden and abrupt change to generic prescribing, without ensuring the quality of generic drugs, can have disastrous results, as the abortive Pakistani experience of 1973 shows. It has to conquer the hostility of the élites who feel their standards of health care threatened, and to counter pressures mounted by the TNCs themselves — all requiring political determination, care and moderation.

If a rationalised list of drugs is adopted, the main focus of policy should be to economise in its provision, subject to two important considerations (besides the crucial one of quality noted above):

(1) It should attempt to promote indigenous industrial and technological development, even if this involves some costs (e.g. technology purchase, R and D investment, tariff protection) in the short run. The pharmaceutical sector, and with it the fine chemicals industry sector, has numerous 'linkages' which are favourable to long-term industrial development, and countries with large markets, a broad industrial base and sufficient skilled manpower can reasonably

attempt to expand into the production of intermediate and basic chemicals required for pharmaceutical manufacture. This is not intended to advocate highly protected 'self-sufficiency' in this industry. It is doubtful, in view of the rapid pace of technological change, whether any country can be fully self-sufficient. But a large degree of local production in countries like India, Brazil, Mexico and Egypt may be feasible and economical. Similarly, R and D should be undertaken selectively and according to comparative advantage. There is a good case for leaving basic R and D and expensive product development to TNCs which are already engaged in it, and to concentrate LDC efforts on process development and adaptation, and perhaps on discovering drugs for tropical diseases not adequately researched by TNCs.

(2) Since the R and D efforts of TNCs in many areas are valuable and desirable, policies to economise on drug purchase *should not curtail their earnings in such a way that desirable R and D is reduced.* It may thus be advisable for LDCs to pay premium prices for genuinely innovative products of TNCs even when cheaper substitutes are available from imitative firms. This leads to the creation of a two-tier price structure, with high-priced innovations and generically priced old products, a structure which is in fact evolving in several advanced countries (most notably France, and, for the Federal-financed health sector, in the US). It must be pointed out, however, that such a price structure raises two further problems: first, LDCs may want a further two-tier division within the innovative drugs themselves, paying less for 'rich man's drugs' which are intended for diseases prevalent in developed countries and more for drugs of major interest to tropical areas;[30] second, TNCs' R and D is financed not simply by innovations but by profits earned on all products, old and new, and cutting down the prices of old products may simply transfer the burden to new ones (if LDCs want mainly old products, this would in effect shift the burden to the developed countries: not an undesirable procedure).

Subject to these considerations, LDCs should try to meet their drug needs from the most economical available sources, local and foreign. The exact method of determining prices (including transfer prices) and rewarding R and D is a complex matter which we cannot discuss here, but a range of alternative systems is in use in different countries to provide models for study. The purchase of drugs on a worldwide tender basis may require some amendment to existing patent laws, but, in view of what has been said about the need to preserve basic research, an abolition of patent protection may not be advisable. On the contrary, some *strengthening* of patents may be required in instances where drug development has become lengthier and more risky. An interesting recent development — perhaps originating in the growth of generic prescribing in the US and the entry of large firms in generic markets in a big way — is the offer of some TNCs to provide older drugs at cost to LDCs via WHO. It is very likely that this will culminate in TNCs explicitly entering the international market for generics and competing with small producers with their older branded products. The result may be anti-competitive (i.e. small firms will not be able to compete even on generic drugs) but not necessarily unwelcome for the LDCs, since this would greatly reduce their 'search costs' for cheap drugs of adequate quality.

(3) Policy reform should encompass the marketing and promotion of drugs. If generic prescribing takes hold, the need for commercial promotion will decline except for new drugs, and governments may wish to institute controls on the cost and content of advertising. Controls may range from mild exhortation on cost, or vetting of advertising, to strict statutory regulation, or even to official takeover of the information function. The provision of adequate information is not, by any means, an easy task. It requires a grid along which full data on new therapies and their relative benefits and costs are effectively communicated to doctors, and along which doctors' findings on efficacy and adverse reactions can be communicated to manufacturers, officials and other parts of the health system. It is likely that an official structure can provide such a grid more economically and with more objectivity than is presently done by the drug companies, but the difficulties of setting-up and administering such a centralised system should not be minimised.

We may conclude on an optimistic note. Most of the reforms recommended here have already been launched in the developed countries, and their experience offers a wealth of lessons to LDCs which wish to minimise the costs of drug provision to their populations. There is a growing awareness of the problems that drug provision in the present structure faces, and the large firms are themselves adapting to the changing pressures and circumstances without great discomfort. The conflict and confrontation which seemed to overshadow the scene a year or two ago[31] seem gradually to be yielding to a spirit of meaningful debate (if not co-operation). The next few years may see major changes in the international system of drug production, pricing and distribution, though it is less likely that the dominance of TNCs will diminish significantly in most areas.

Notes

1. This chapter has benefited greatly from the comments and criticisms of several experts, but it retains a number of points on which they may disagree. I hope that, despite this, Jorge Katz, Alan Maislisch and Erich Kaufer will accept my thanks. I wish to acknowledge my gratitude, in particular, to Andrew Herxheimer for his patience and encouragement.

2. For a selection of recent works see Schwartzman (1976) and Reekie (1975).

3. See Grabowski and Vernon (1976) and Schnee and Caglarcan (1976).

4. Grabowski and Vernon (1976).

5. This discussion relies mainly on evidence for the US and may not apply to the same extent to the European countries, where generic competition is not as advanced.

6. In the UK, greater levels of competition may also be due to increasing penetration by foreign pharmaceutical companies (especially from Europe) in recent years.

7. See Schwartzman (1976), Teeling-Smith (1979) and Grabowski and Vernon (1976).

8. For US figures see Schwartzman (1976) and for the UK figures see Slatter (1977).

9. See Cooper and Cooper (1972).

10. This is argued by OHE (1975) and Reekie (1977). For a critique, and evidence from Sri Lanka on persisting price differences, see Lall (1978b).

11. See Slatter (1977) and Schwartzman (1976).

12. Schwartzman (1976) argues that if R and D were capitalised, the rate of profit would be reduced significantly: however, this only occurs if the rate at which R and D is depreciated exceeds new R and D greatly, and it is not clear how justified this assumption is. Moreover, it clearly makes tax sense to treat R and D as a current expense, since this is how company accountants prefer to treat it.

13. See Lall (1973).

14. *Scrip*, 19 November, 1977, 2. The classic case of transfer pricing in Europe is in the UK, by Hoffman La Roche, for diazepam and chlordiazepoxide; see the Monopolies Commission (1973).

15. See Bibile (1977), Lall and Bibile (1977).

16. Slatter (1977). After a detailed analysis of product introductions, sales and promotion, he concludes that 'The required levels of promotional expenditure act as significant barriers to market entry . . . The mean for all ten classes (of drugs with high promotional expenditures) was £249,000, an increase of 111 per cent over the mean level in 1968' (p. 85).

17. On Latin America see Ledogar (1975) and Silverman (1976). The latter shows that there is far greater intensity of drug representatives per doctor in poor countries of Latin America than in the US.

18. *Scrip*, November 5th, 1977, 22.

19. Ibid., 23.

20. India has reduced the life of drug patents to 7 years. Italy and Brazil do not permit patents on drug products or processes, though Italy has now adopted

a legal device which in effect recognises patents. A number of LDCs, e.g. Argentina, interpret the law liberally in order to favour domestic enterprises which infringe foreign patents. In developed countries, on the other hand, the tendency is to strengthen patent protection; the UK has extended patent coverage from 17 to 20 years.

21. See Slatter (1977).

22. For a discussion of these in the case of Sri Lanka see Lall and Bibile (1977).

23. This was noted for India by the Hathi Committee (1975).

24. Tests by the FDA found that 40-60 per cent of ethical drugs, and, from a sample of 420 over-the-counter drugs, 75 per cent of non-ethical drugs, lacked evidence of effectiveness. Hundreds of drugs withdrawn from the US market continue to be sold in other countries. Ledogar (1975) and Silverman (1976) find that several drugs in the high toxicity range were being sold in Latin America after being banned in the US and Europe.

25. The Summit Meeting of the Non-Aligned Nations in 1976 endorsed a programme of comprehensive reform of the pharmaceutical industry; this is now being explored by a joint task force of WHO, UNCTAD and UNIDO. In response, some major European TNCs have offered to provide a number of essential drugs at cost to the Third World via the WHO.

26. A lengthier discussion is provided in Lall (1978a).

27. See Segall (1975) for a detailed explanation.

28. *Scrip*, 12 November 1977, 16. The International Federation of Pharmaceutical Manufacturers' Associations has, predictably, 'strongly opposed' the concept of an essential drug list on medical and economic grounds, and argued that such a list would lead to worsening of health care standards.

29. For a detailed description of the rationalisation in Sri Lanka see Bibile (1977) and for the problems in implementing the reform see Lall and Bibile (1977).

30. This is argued in Lall (1978a), where I also note that any scheme of pricing which discriminates between countries is likely to run into severe difficulties with governments which are asked to pay high prices. Thus, such a scheme would require tripartite agreement between the TNCs, the LDCs and the developed countries − politically a rather unlikely outcome.

31. The violent reaction of the TNCs to my (1975) study illustrates this clearly; three separate monographs were issued attacking this study, and the US PMA publicly denounced it (see *Scrip*, 13 December 1975, 2). Many of the reforms recommended there now seem acceptable or even in force, and the offer of cheap drugs by TNCs is a major admission of the inequities of the present pricing system.

References

Bibile, S. (1977). *Pharmaceutical Policies in Sri Lanka*, Geneva, UNCTAD, TD/B/C.6/21

Brooke, P.A. (1975). *Resistant Prices: A Study of Competitive Strains in the Antibiotic Markets*, New York, Council of Economic Priorities

Coleman, V. (1975). *The Medicine Men*, London, Temple Smith

Cooper, M.H. and Cooper, A.J. (1972). *International Price Comparisons*, London, National Economic Development Office

Cox, J.S.G., Millane, B.V. and Styles, A.E.J. (1975). A planning model of pharmaceutical research and development. *R and D Management*, June

Grabowski, H.G. and Vernon, J.M. (1976). Structural effects of regulation on innovation in the ethical drug industry. In Masson, R.J. and Qualls, P.D. (eds.), *Essays in Industrial Organisation*, Cambridge (Mass), Ballinger

Hathi Committee (1975). *Report of the Committee on Drugs and Pharmaceuticals Industry*, New Delhi, Ministry of Petroleum and Chemicals

Lall, S. (1973). Transfer pricing by multinational manufacturing firms, *Oxford Bulletin of Economics and Statistics*

—— (1974). The international pharmaceutical industry and less developed countries with special reference to India, *Oxford Bulletin of Economics and Statistics*

—— (1975). *Major Issues in Transfer of Technology to Developing Countries: A Case Study of the Pharmaceutical Industry*, Geneva, UNCTAD, TD/B/C.6/4

—— (1978a). *The Growth of the Pharmaceutical Industry in Developing Countries. Problems and Prospects*, UNIDO, Vienna, ID/204

—— (1978b). Price competition and the international pharmaceutical industry, *Oxford Bulletin of Economics and Statistics*, February

Lall, S. and Bibile, S. (1977). The political economy or controlling transnationals: the pharmaceutical industry in Sri Lanka (1972-76), *World Development*, August

Ledogar, R.J. (1975). *Hungry for Profits*, New York, IDOC/North America

Monopolies Commission (1973). *Chlordiazepoxide and Diazepam*, London, HMSO

OHE (1975). *The Canberra Hypothesis*, London, Office of Health Economics

Reekie, W.D. (1975). *The Economics of the Pharmaceutical Industry*, London, Macmillan

—— (1977). *Pricing New Pharmaceutical Products*, London, Croom Helm

Rucker, T.D. (1973). Economic aspects of drug over use, *Medical Annals of the District of Columbia*, December

Schnee, J. and Caglarcan, E. (1976). The changing pharmaceutical R and D environment, *Business Economics*, May

Schwartzman, D. (1976). *Innovation in the Pharmaceutical Industry*, Baltimore, Johns Hopkins

Segall, M. (1975). Pharmaceuticals and health planning in developing countries, Sussex, Institute of Development Studies, Communication 119

Silverman, M. (1976). *The Drugging of the Americas*, Berkeley, University of California Press

Slatter, S.S.P. (1977). *Competition and Marketing Strategies in the Pharmaceutical Industry*, London, Croom Helm

Teeling-Smith, G. (ed.) (1979). *Medicines for the Year 2000*, London, Office of Health Economics

8 THE ROLE OF INTERNATIONAL ORGANISATIONS IN MEDICINES POLICY

Catherine Stenzl

A number of international organisations are directly or indirectly
concerned with the provision and use of medicines. Apart from the
organisations which take an explicit interest in medicines policy,
organisations concerned with trade, development issues or population
problems can have an impact by regulating trade, or by influencing
priorities or resources in drug supply. It is not possible in a short
chapter to describe or analyse the activities of all these agencies.
We concentrate on some of the key organisations directly concerned
in medicines policy, those in the field of regulation, promoting
production and distribution systems.

We will first examine the organisation within the UN system which
has an explicit mandate to deal with drug issues, i.e. the World Health
Organisation. The development of WHO policy since the early sixties
illustrates the changing perspective of the international community
in this field and provides a view of how policies develop within the
system.

In the area of drug production the United Nations Industrial
Development Organisation (UNIDO) has been playing an active role.
After a brief description of its work we will summarise the main points
of the overall approach which for the last five years has been emerging
in the UN system.

As an example of a regional organisation we will then briefly look
at the medicines policy of the European Community. Other regional
organisations play an active role in medicines policy: the Pan American
Health Organisation, the Council of Europe, EFTA and others. The
EEC is an important example because it represents an area of considerable pharmaceuticals production and consumption and because
– unlike other organisations – it can legislate directly for its member
states.

Two areas which are related to medicines policy are not covered
in this chapter: contraception and control of psychoactive substances.
Population control, or fertility management as it is called in the
international jargon, has become a high priority in the work of many
international organisations. UNIDO called it the 'most singly

important world problem' (ID/WG 116/14, p. 1). More and more agencies are working out programmes in this field, more and more funds have been made available (WHO research funds for fertility control for instance increased from 30,000 dollars in 1963 to 4.5 million dollars in 1972). Since the lack of health care infrastructures in developing countries makes it difficult to distribute contraceptives through the medical system, it is sometimes recommended (e.g. in ID/WG 116/16, p. 20) that mechanical and chemical contraceptives – which are in many countries considered as drugs – should be distributed and marketed more like non-drug items.

The argument behind such recommendations is that the consequences of a lack of contraception are more serious than the consequences of the distribution of contraceptives without the medical supervision which is possible and considered necessary in industrialised countries. In view of the wide application of population programmes and considering the reservations of some health authorities (e.g. in the USA and UK) against certain injectable contraceptives which are proposed to developing countries, a thorough study on how the medical and social implications of such programmes are assessed might be both useful and necessary.

International efforts in the control of psychoactive substances were thoroughly analysed in a very interesting study, Bruun *et al.* (1975), updated in 1978 (Pan and Bruun, 1979). The fact that a growing number of therapeutic drugs have become objects of illicit trade and non-medical use illustrates the close relation between this problem and medicines policy. A study of the complex area between, on the one hand, illicit trade in and use of such substances and, on the other hand, their medical use – the rationality of which has sometimes been questioned – might produce some recommendations on how the problem could be dealt within in a wider framework than that of the control of production and international commerce. The general policy problem of international drug control has been addressed in the UNSDRI publication, Controlling Drugs (Blum, Bovet and Moore, 1974).

The UN System

The World Health Organisation is one of the specialised agencies of the United Nations system. Its objective is the 'attainment by all peoples of the highest possible level of health' (Constitution, art. 1), health being defined as 'a state of complete physical, mental and social wellbeing and not merely absence of disease or infirmity' (Constitution, preamble). According to the Constitution, WHO, in order to achieve its aim, acts as the directing and co-ordinating authority on international health work, provides assistance in strengthening health services, promotes work and co-operation in the eradication of diseases and in the advancement of health in general, provides information, promotes research and training, establishes international nomenclatures of diseases and public health practices and sets standards with respect to food, biological and pharmaceutical products. It can propose conventions, agreements and regulations and make recommendations with regard to international health matters.

Membership is open to states, whether or not they are members of the United Nations; WHO is funded by contributions from member states according to a scale of assessment derived from the UN scale, which is based on a country's population and gross national product. In 1979 there were 153 members and associate members. The largest contributions were paid by: USA 25 per cent, Soviet Union 13.34 per cent (this includes the contributions from Ukrania, Byelorussia and Mongolia, which are always listed separately), Japan 8.5 per cent, Federal Republic of Germany 7.58 per cent, France 5.73 per cent, China 5.41 per cent. The UK, Italy, Canada, Australia, Spain, Netherlands, Poland, German Democratic Republic, Sweden, Belgium and Brazil contributed (in order of decreasing contributions) between 4.45 per cent and 1 per cent; all the other 133 members paid less than 1 per cent of the WHO budget (WHO 32.8).

The World Health Assembly, which meets once a year (less frequent meetings are under consideration), determines the policy of WHO, names the 30 member states which will be represented on the Executive Board and appoints the Director-General who heads the Secretariat.

Article 21 of the Constitution states that

the Health Assembly shall have authority to adopt regulations concerning . . .
(d) standards with respect to the safety, purity and potency of biological, pharmaceutical and similar products moving in international commerce
(e) advertising and labelling of biologial, pharmaceutical and similar products moving in international commerce.

This specific authority to deal with medicines is complemented by Article 23, which gives the Assembly a general authority to deal with health questions. The possibility of adopting binding regulations has so far never been used.

During the first ten years of its existence WHO's concern with medicines was essentially limited to quality control in terms of the chemical and physical properties of drugs. The standardisation of biological substances, the setting of specifications for pharmaceutical products in the International Pharmacopoeia (WHO inherited both these programmes from the League of Nations) and later the work on international non-proprietary names for drugs were designed to improve international quality control. Around 1960 the discussion on drug safety and efficacy began within the organisation, but it took the contergan/thalidomide events to shock WHO into action (Off. Rec. 144, p. 301). Following a Swedish initiative the 15th Assembly adopted in May 1962 a resolution (WHA 15.41) requesting a feasibility study to see whether WHO could establish minimum basic requirements and recommend standard methods for the clinical and pharmaceutical evaluation of medicines, organise a regular exchange of information on safety and efficacy and secure prompt transmission to national health authorities of new information on serious side effects of pharmaceutical preparations.

One sees from the records (Official Records, *119*, Committee on Programme and Budget, 14th and 15th meeting) that the paragraph on exchange of information on safety and efficacy which became the first proposal to be at least partially implemented was the most controversial one. The German and later the French delegation wanted it deleted altogether on the grounds that it would place on WHO a responsibility that it could not fulfil without serious risk. Even after the original wording 'WHO should promote international exchange of information' had been weakened to read only that ways and means for such an exchange should be studied, there were nevertheless lengthy discussions and a number of amendments before the text was adopted.

One year later the Assembly requested member states to communicate to WHO (who would then pass on the information to all members) immediately any decision to prohibit or limit availability of a drug already in use, any decision to refuse approval of a new drug and any approval for general use of a new drug when accompanied by restrictive provisions; this request was limited by the sentence 'if these decisions are taken as a result of serious adverse reactions' (WHA 16.36).

Indeed the field of adverse reactions was for a few years to remain the main issue on which new action was visibly and relatively quickly taken. The same resolution of 1963 invited member states systematically to collect information on adverse reactions, and the possibility of setting up an international monitoring system of adverse reactions was studied. In 1965 the American government offered facilities for the processing of information on adverse drug reactions, a pilot project was carried out with the help of these facilities and an American grant led eventually to the creation of the WHO Drug Monitoring Centre in 1972. This monitoring system relies on information transmitted by national centres. It can only be as effective as the information it receives. The difficulties in collecting such information on a national level are indicated in Chapter 5, p. 97. By 1975, 21 national centres were participating in the scheme which had by then received 101,775 reports concerning 9700 drug names.

Quality control and surveillance of safety and efficacy of drugs raise particular problems for developing countries which have few or no facilities for drug control and are heavily dependent on imported medicines. An awareness of these difficulties — at least as far as chemical and physical quality is concerned — is visible in some technical reports (e.g. The Use of Specifications for Pharmaceutical Properties, T.R. 138, 1957 and The Quality Control of Pharmaceutical Preparations, T.R. 249, 1961) and in the organisation of a training programme in quality control. On a worldwide level the Assembly approached the problem in two ways:

(1) by asking that WHO study ways and means of offering advice and assistance to member states in developing their own facilities or helping them to gain access to facilities in other countries;
(2) by requesting the Executive Board to examine ways and means of ensuring that drugs exported from a producing country comply with the drug control requirements which apply in that country for domestic use (WHA 16.36).

Later resolutions show quite clearly that this second principle was not easily applied: in January 1967 the Executive Board expressed its concern that such requests to member states were not yet generally applied (EB 39.RB). WHO began drafting principles for quality control procedures which should be included in good manufacturing practice. In 1968 the Assembly requested the inclusion of a certification scheme on the quality of pharmaceutical products in international commerce

(WHA 21.37). The requirements for 'Good practices in the manufacture and quality control of drugs' and the certification scheme were adopted in 1969 (WHA 22.50) and three years later the Director-General was able to report that quite a number of countries were applying or considering to apply these texts.[1] In 1977 a list of countries which applied the certification scheme was published in the WHO Chronicle (*31*, 12, annex).[2] Two important drug-producing countries, the Federal Republic of Germany and Switzerland, are conspicuous by their absence from the list. They explain their non-participation by citing legal difficulties arising from their federal structure. At present, WHO is trying to solve these legal problems.

After the Thalidomide events it would have been difficult for anyone to object to or to delay action on adverse drug reactions. The general problem of safety and efficacy, however, raised more difficulties. It was discussed several times at the Assembly and a number of expert groups studied aspects of the issue.[3] In 1970 the Assembly widened the information scheme set up in 1963 to include any decision to withdraw or restrict availability of a drug already in use if the decision was taken because of lack of substantial evidence of effectiveness in relation to the drug's toxicity and the purpose for which it is used (WHA 23.48). One year later the Director-General was asked to consider the creation of a system of collection and dissemination of information on results of safety and effectiveness trials of new drugs and their registration in countries having the necessary facilities, so that these data might possibly be used by the health authorities of countries importing pharmaceutical products (WHA 24.56). The same resolution underlined the importance of an overall approach to questions relating to pharmacology and drug control. It demonstrates a considerable evolution from the original compartmentalised approach — when pharmaceutical quality control was discussed quite separately from safety and efficacy — to a much more integrated view of the problem. This change fits into an overall trend within WHO away from a mainly technical approach focusing on the eradication of specific diseases to a more comprehensive one which sees health not only in a medical but also in a social and economic context.

This changing approach goes hand in hand with efforts to decentralise WHO work to bring it into closer contact with effective health needs of member states and with an increasing awareness of the problems of developing countries. It was formally decided in 1976 that WHO should give priority to the concerns of developing countries.

Economic considerations begin to appear in the texts and the report on WHO's work in 1970 (Official Records, 180, p. 51-53) mentions co-operation with UNIDO in planning the establishment of pharmaceutical industries in developing countries, a theme taken up with some emphasis in 1978, when the Assembly declared that the local production of essential drugs and vaccines is a 'legitimate aspiration' of developing countries and it requests co-operation with other agencies in order to assist countries in establishing local production corresponding to their health needs 'it being understood that financing should be independent of the source of technology' (WHA 31.32); these two sentences give some indication of the difficulties experienced in this field (see Lall, 1978). A new sub-programme on drug policies and management was launched in 1975 when the Assembly underlined the necessity of developing drug policies linking drug research, production and distribution with real health needs (WHA 28.66) — an issue which was also the subject of a technical discussion in 1976. This new approach led to the drafting of a model list of essential drugs which was published in a technical report in 1977 together with recommendations on provision of minimum information on medicine use and effect for prescribers. The action programme on essential drugs (WHA 31.32) urges member states to establish procurement, storage and distribution systems in order to make available drugs of adequate quality at reasonable prices; to establish national drug lists; to enact legislation for drug registration, use and control. It also requests that WHO improve its supply services, encourage local production in co-operation with other agencies, study ways of reducing drug prices and promote the development of quality control systems.

The reports and records of the first years of work on the clinical aspects of medicines leave the observer with the impression that a very cautious and somewhat hesitant secretariat was pushed into action by the Assembly. The report of a scientific group on the safety and efficacy of drugs which was drafted in early 1963 was never published and remains to this day restricted for internal use only. We understand that it contains quite clear recommendations on the need for an exchange of information in the area of drug testing and on safety and efficacy of new drugs, as well as an appeal urgently to establish a service providing worldwide information on serious adverse drug reactions. The Director-General, however, reported only on the issue of safety and efficacy, saying that the group thought that an invitation to member states to furnish data in relation to drugs which have been approved or rejected 'might be appropriate' (Official Records, 127, p. 167). In 1967 the Director-General reported that a certification scheme for drugs moving in international commerce was not feasible at that time (A20/P+B/10, p. 2) – an attitude criticised by the Norwegian delegate as defeatist (Official Records, 161, p. 274). The Director-General's negativism was promptly disregarded by the Assembly, who requested the setting up of the scheme (WHA 21.37).

In spite of the Secretariat's hesitations, the published WHO reports describing the agency's work in the sixties paint a picture of considerable activity which is not always supported by facts. WHO reports were, therefore, misleading. One example: the organisational chart of the secretariat attached to the Director-General's report (Official Records, 139, annex 8) gives the impression that by 1965 a new unit 'Pharmacology and Toxicology' had been created in the relevant division.[4] According to the programme-budget this unit consists of seven staff members. A closer look at the tasks of this unit, however, shows that it is none other than the old unit for addiction-producing drugs which had been entrusted with the implementation of the early resolutions with a corresponding increase of staff from four to seven in 1963. The budget figures of that time show that the proportion of WHO headquarter and interregional resources spent on drug work remained fairly constant (see Tables 8.1, 8.2 and 8.3).

From 1971 drug expenditure increases, both in absolute figures and as a proportion of total headquarters' and interregional activities. This increase was entirely used to finance the operating costs for the monitoring programme for adverse reactions, with a concurrent fall in expenditure proportion for other drug-related activities as the monitoring programme expanded. From 1979 the operating costs of the programme (which will be transferred to Uppsala) will be borne by Sweden and the proportion of drug work in interregional funds drops back to the level of 1967. Headquarter expenditure, however, has been rising steadily since 1975, a trend which is confirmed in the percentages indicated in the latest programme-budget, where drug division expenditure is related to total expenditure (see Table 8.4). The transfer of the monitoring programme also means that the staff funds of that programme can now be used for increasing the staff working in other tasks in the unit for drug policy and management.

Considering that drug expenditure can amount to 10-20 per cent of health expenditure in developed countries and to 40-60 per cent in developing countries (Science and Technology for Health Promotion

Table 8.1: Programme-Budget; Headquarters Programme Activities (Expressed in Dollars)

	1961	1963	1965	1967	1969	1971	1973	1975	1977	1979
Biological Standardisation	39,833	58,404	44,318	45,790	51,966	56,221	47,880	120,568	140,720	242,800
Pharmaceuticals	47,926	55,984	58,435	67,808	78,398	88,227	85,253	175,321	231,490	
Drug Safety and Efficacy		23,248	34,571	91,350	101,544	47,201	47,494	242,697	263,070	1,001,200
Drug Monitoring						54,062	55,877			
Director's Office	8,184	17,303	13,963	21,691	30,816	32,055	112,204	132,746	173,440	240,800
Total	95,943	154,979	151,287	266,639	262,724	277,766	348,708	671,332	808,720	1,484,800
Total Headquarters programme activities	4,228,689	6,285,949	7,261,465	10,845,769	13,040,685	15,481,605	18,130,749	19,759,704	24,471,275	33,017,800
Percentage of drug work of total HQ programmes	2.2%	2.4%	2%	2.4%	2%	1.8%	1.9%	3.4%	3.3%	4.5%
Number of staff in medicines work	14	17	17	24	24	24	24	23	23	33

A varying number of units with changing names were part of the division Biology and Pharmacology. In our calculations we did not include the units for drug dependence, immunology and food additives which were at times part of the division, unless they were doing work in medicines policy as such. For 1963 for instance we calculated the figure for safety and efficacy as 3/7 of the figure for the drug dependence unit which had its staff increased from 4 to 7 when it was asked to implement resolution WHA 15.41. in 1967 the proportion was taken into account is 10/13 of the unit which was by then renamed Pharmacology and Toxicology.
   The figure for the Director's Office was calculated as the proportion of the total figure corresponding to the proportion of division funds allocated to the relevant units.
   From 1977 the staff figures are expressed in man-hours. From 1973 costs for consultants and travel are included in the figures for the Director's Office and no longer under individual units.
   From 1975 the new budget presentation does not single out programme activities in the same way. In order to get comparable figures we calculated our figure for total headquarter programme activities on the basis of the same items previously included under that category.
   The staff increase in 1979 is due to the transfer of staff from the monitoring programme to headquarter units.

Source: WHO Official Records, Programme Budgets.

Table 8.2: Programme-Budget; Interregional Activities

	1961	1963	1965	1967	1969	1971	1973	1975	1977	1979
Biological Standardisation		54,480	61,980	78,500	88,500	98,000	98,600	74,100	74,500	84,500
Pharmaceuticals		7,800	12,000	17,500	19,000	20,000	20,000	15,000	17,250	26,000
Drug Safety and Efficacy			25,000	10,000	10,000	10,000	13,000	9,750	12,250	
Drug Monitoring				20,000	20,000	20,000	20,000	15,000	15,000	121,300
Monitoring Programme for adverse reactions						345,000	378,312	562,818	487,640	
Total		62,280	98,980	126,000	137,500	493,000	529,912	676,668	606,640	231,800
Total interregional activities		3,527,707	4,409,064	5,260,847	6,828,253	7,622,274	8,809,323	10,287,875	10,311,665	9,690,300
Percentage of medicines work		1.76%	2.24%	2.39%	2.01%	6.46%	6.01%	6.57%	5.88%	2.39%
% without monitoring progr.						1.94%	1.72%	1.11%	1.05%	
Permanent staff (all in monitoring programme)						18	17	17	12	1

Since we are interested in the general trend, we included only those programmes which appear for more than two consecutive years and therefore represent an on-going commitment.

The monitoring programme for adverse reactions represents a major financial effort. In order to give a clearer picture of expenditure for medicines programmes we indicate the figure for this programme separately and calculated the percentage figure for medicines work both including and excluding this programme. From 1979 the operating costs for the programme are financed by Sweden and therefore no longer appear in the programme budget.

Table 8.3: Programme-Budget: Summary of Headquarters and Interregional Activities

	1963	1965	1967	1969	1971	1973	1975	1977	1979
Headquarters and inter-regional medicine-related activities	217,259	250,267	392,639	400,224	770,766	878,620	1,348,000	1,415,360	1,716,600
Total headquarters and inter-regional activities	9,813,656	11,670,529	16,106,616	19,869,038	23,103,879	26,940,072	30,047,579	34,099,790	42,708,100
Percentage of medicine-related work	2.21%	2.14%	2.43%	2.01%	3.33%	3.26%	4.48%	4.15%	4.01%
% without monitoring programme					1.84%	1.86%	2.61%	2.72%	

Table 8.4: Expenditure on the division Prophylactic and Therapeutic Substances (previously Pharmacology and Toxicology)

	1976	1977	1978	1979
Proportion of the regular budget allocated to the division	2.6% (1.6%)	3.4% (2.3%)	2.9% (1.8%)	3% (2%)
Proportion of total expenditure	2.2% (1%)	2.7% (1.4%)	2.1% (1.2%)	2.09% (1.4%)

The figures in brackets show the expenditure without the unit Health Laboratory Services, which was previously part of the division Strengthening of Health Services and was moved to Prophylactic and Therapeutic Substances in 1974. This unit is not included in the figures in Table 8.1.

Source: WHO Official Records, Programme-Budgets.

in Developing Countries, WHO document for the UN Conference on Science and Technology for Development, 1979), the proportion of WHO funds allocated to drug-related work seems more than modest for a programme which aims at giving advice and assistance in establishing comprehensive drug policies, carrying out research and running information systems on a worldwide level. Compared with industry expenditure on promotion of drugs, which is estimated at 2,700 million dollars in 1974 for 34 leading firms alone,[5] WHO resources are minute.

Until the early seventies WHO's work was essentially an attempt to harmonise drug standards in international commerce: the emphasis lies on quality control — first in terms of chemical and physical properties, later also in terms of clinical quality. The exchange of information on adverse reactions and drug registration attempts to make this control more effective on a worldwide level. The not very extensive work on advertising belongs in the same area. After a first resolution in 1952 (WHA 5,76) which warned against the advertising of new drugs as 'wonder' or 'miracle' drugs, and apart from a survey of legislation in the International Digest of Health Legislation in 1963 (updated in 1968) little was done until 1968 when WHO published the 'Ethical and Scientific criteria for Pharmaceutical Advertising' which include a list of information which should appear in all advertising[6] and restricts advertising to the general public to a limited range of OTC (over-the-counter) drugs (WHA 21.41).

From the early seventies onward the reports indicate a change in policy as well as in style. The secretariat appears to play a more active role and to take a more concrete and detailed interest in the needs of member countries. The emphasis shifts from the regulation of existing trade to the more fundamental question of what drugs are needed where, and how these needs can best be met with available resources. In his detailed report of 1975 (Official Records 226, annex 13) the Director-General underlines the need for research in drug use, for assessment of drug needs and for evaluation of methods in pharmaceutical marketing. The action programme for essential drugs in 1978 confirms the reorientation from the regulation of commerce to more specifically problem- and aid-oriented work.

Political and economic influences are not absent from work at the international level. A programme which explicitly states that the concerns of developing countries must come first, and which at least implicitly questions the present economic and decision-making structures in provision and use of medicines, might – if implemented – have a considerable impact on vested interests, commercial, political or ideological. The decision of the US Congress that field work should in future only be supported on a bilateral basis and no longer through the general funds of international organisations seems to be a reaction to the positions and demands articulated by developing countries in WHO and elsewhere, and to the international organisation's apparent responsiveness to such demands. This and the fact that the Director-General calls the subject of pharmaceutical industries in developing countries a 'minefield' and repeatedly calls for political support for the action programme (A31/12) indicate that the programme was not adopted without opposition and is not expected to be implemented without difficulties.

Whereas WHO's earlier approach to drug problems was essentially technical, medical, and therefore clearly and more or less exclusively within WHO's competence and mandate, the present policy with emphasis on the social and economic aspects of drug issues has wider implications and connects more directly with the programmes of other UN agencies, in particular UNIDO and to a certain extent UNCTAD. Both these organisations emerged in the sixties in the wake of the UN's increasing preoccupation with problems of development, industrialisation and trade.

UNIDO (United Nations Industrial Development Organisation), set up to deal with industrialisation, was formally established at the beginning of 1967 and is part of the UN Secretariat. At the moment efforts are being made to transform it into a fully fledged specialised agency within the UN system. Its tasks are described in the founding resolution of the UN General Assembly (Resolution 2152) as follows:

> to carry out surveys of possibilities for industrialisation;
> to give assistance in efficient utilisation of industrial capacities;
> to give assistance in developing and improving market and distribution techniques and in the development of export-oriented industries;
> to give assistance in training of personnel;
> to give assistance in dissemination of information on technological innovations and know-how;
> to give assistance in establishing or strengthening institutions . . . including applied research, standardisation and quality control.

The technical assistance which is the core of UNIDO's field work is financed from various sources within the UN budget (the UN Development Programme is an important source) and through voluntary government contributions.

The pharmaceutical industry became quite soon an area of interest, and in 1969 UNIDO convened an expert working group on the establishment of pharmaceutical industries in developing countries which examined the questions of quality control and training of personnel, analysed the economic and technological aspects of the issue and recommended the assessment of therapeutic needs, so that production could be developed in the context of these needs; it also pointed out that the most urgently needed drugs might not necessarily be the most profitable ones to produce (ID/35). In spite of such recommendations UNIDO's programmes during those first years were very much concentrated 'on the technical aspects – establishing plants, improving facilities, training specialists' (ID/204, p. 40) and expected productions in developing countries to develop and grow within the existing structures of medicine supply. It took some time until wider considerations began to appear not only as one aspect but as a fundamental criterion for programmes. In 1975 the International Consultation Meeting in the Field of Pharmaceutical Industries in Budapest prepared a tentative list of essential drugs[7] and in later papers, particularly the ones from the Second Panel of Experts on the Pharmaceutical Industry in 1978 (ID/WG 267) it is said clearly that the drugs produced or imported have to be 'related to prevailing disease patterns and economic conditions of the country' (ID/WG/ 267/1), and that the preparation of a list of essential drugs is therefore the first step to be taken in any effort to promote the growth of pharmaceutical industries in developing countries. It is also suggested that drug registration and quality control should be harmonised on a regional level between countries with similar conditions and that indigenous systems of medicines should be used in conjunction with Western medicine. A further working group examined the possibility of drug production from medicinal plants (ID/WG.271). Following the 'Lima Declaration' of 1975 which calls for a larger share in the world's industrial production for developing countries, UNIDO started to organise a number of sectorial consultations between developing and industrialised countries to explore the possibilities for achieving this goal. In early 1979 a preparatory meeting for the consultation in the pharmaceutical sector stated clearly that developing countries should not 'imitate the pattern of supply in developed countries where different products are sold in different combinations and dosage forms' and recommended that an 'integrated development of the entire system of procurement, production and distribution of pharmaceuticals at the national level appears the best way' to achieve the objective of concentrating production on the essential drugs required to meet health care needs (ID/WG. 292/3, p. 5). The need for a new framework for international co-operation in developing the pharmaceutical industry is underlined with particular emphasis on co-operation between developing countries. The meeting also suggests that the consultation should address itself to the possibility of establishing 'guidelines for licensing agreements for the transfer of technology for basic manufacture of the active ingredients of essential drugs' and calls for an increase in contributions to the UN Industrial Development Fund and the UN Development Programme, so that the Fund could acquire technology for the production of essential drugs on behalf of the developing countries.

A similar approach appears in a number of studies published by UNCTAD, in which the problems relating to the transfer of technology in the pharmaceutical industry are analysed. One of these studies (Lall and UNCTAD, 1975) suggested the establishment of regional co-operative centres for pharmaceutical production and technology, an idea taken up by the Fifth Conference of Heads of State or Government of Non-Aligned Countries (Colombo 1976) and endorsed by the Group of 77 in Mexico later in the same year. The Colombo resolution led to the establishment of a joint task force between UNIDO, WHO and UNCTAD,[8] which with the assistance of the UN Development Programme is to give the technical advice necessary for the implementation of the resolution within the framework of the UN Action Programme for Economic Cooperation (UNAPEC). The Colombo resolution also called for the establishment of national agencies for the purchase of pharmaceuticals at reasonable prices so that they could act as a 'temporary catalyst'. UNICEF, an organisation entirely financed by voluntary contributions, is involved in this particular area of drug procurement: it buys essential drugs in bulk and resells them to developing countries at prices considerably below market prices. In 1977 UNICEF spent 8 million dollars on drugs, out of a total purchases programme for 87 million dollars. According to a UN report (UN 1979) the establishment of a single UN drug purchasing agency for all programmes was proposed in 1977, but so far this proposal has not been followed up.

With the reorientation of WHO and UNIDO programmes and to some extent UNICEF's interest in primary health care, an overall policy for the provision of medicines is emerging from the UN system. Its main elements are:

(1) The needs of developing countries have priority.

(2) Provision of medicines on all levels must be based on real health needs, and integrated into the health care system as a whole.

(3) In order to ensure a production which is appropriate for the local situation, in order to stimulate industrial development and training of personnel, and for economic reasons, the development of pharmaceutical industries in developing countries must be promoted. Depending on the level of industrialisation, units for repackaging, production from intermediate substances, production of active substances and research and development units should be set up.

(4) National and/or regional pharmaceutical centres should be established to deal with purchase of drugs and ingredients, to ensure quality control and drug registration, to train personnel, to carry out research and possibly to act as a model for other functions.

(5) Co-operation among developing countries is essential: sharing of facilities, joint purchase agencies, joint production and the harmonisation of drug registration and control procedures on a regional level can ensure an economic use of resources.

(6) Co-operation between developed and developing countries and with transnational corporations is particularly important in the area of transfer of technology.

(7) The rational use of medicinal plants and indigenous medicine is to be encouraged.

The problems to be tackled by this approach are complex. 'They range from the strictly technological problems common to most industries of obtaining know-how held by companies in developed countries and of fostering indigenous innovation, to the economic difficulties of reducing the costs of buying technology and products in highly imperfect and oligopolistic markets, the medical difficulties of ensuring rational and effective therapeutic practice, the social difficulties of providing for the basic health needs of large numbers of poor people, the legal difficulties of defining property rights, contracts and obligations in the context of the international operations of private firms, and the political difficulties of countering abuses in the present system, with its entrenched interests, by careful and well-directed policies' (Lall 1978, p. 1).

The UN system's new approach to medicines policy has to be seen in the political context of the policy-making bodies of this system, the General Assemblies, where the developing countries hold a majority of the votes which they are increasingly using in order to articulate their specific needs. This constellation is reflected in many resolutions. The adoption of a resolution, however, does not automatically lead to its implementation; in the field of medicines the realisation of many proposals depends to a large extent on the willingness of developed countries, and often their industries, to provide funds and technology. Nor is the voting and implementing of resolutions a simple matter of voting arithmetics. Bruun, Pan and Rexed (1975) describe in some detail how individual countries and various pressure groups exercise or try to exercise their influence in international drug control. Their findings are relevant in our field too: not only are the mechanics of wielding influence – through personal relations, composition of delegations, trade-offs between various areas similar, but many of the actors in the play are the same – the pharmaceutical industry, countries with economic and/or ideological interests, groups with professional interests, etc. The United States' new policy of financing projects only on a bilateral and no longer on a multilateral level appears as an attempt at regaining influence lost to the voting majorities in General Assemblies. Earlier events illustrated by a former head of WHO's division of Pharmacology and Toxicology, who was a paid consultant for them, joining a Swiss pharmaceutical firm, or WHO's granting of official relations to the International Federation of Pharmaceutical Manufacturers' Associations as a non-governmental organisation in 1971 – a decision taken against the recommendations of the competent commission – fit in with the Secretariat's reluctant attitude towards medicines control in the late sixties and early seventies. The pharmaceutical industry has been a growth industry with a strongly multinational form of organisation. The industries' concern over UN policies recommending controls, promoting lists of a necessarily very limited number of essential drugs, or promoting the setting up of independent local industries in developing countries, etc. is obvious. Its countervailing influence is, however, difficult to evaluate.

Although WHO and UNIDO often emphasise the importance of a dialogue and co-operation with the pharmaceutical industry, there is little data available which allows one to assess the form or the content of that dialogue. It is known that in 1977 some manufacturers approached WHO with a proposal to sell a limited number of essential drugs at cost to developing countries in return for recognition of brand names and patents by those countries (ID/204 and UN, 1979). Pending WHO's reply the proposal has not yet been implemented (summer 1979). Apart from this the reports are silent on such contacts. (When the IFPMA representatives were asked to give the industries' point of view in a World Health Assembly, they said that they would prefer to reply through the Secretariat.) A less secretive approach to co-operation between organisations and the industry could contribute to a better view of the problems and possibilities. It would also allow one to form a clearer idea of the significance of allegations such as 'the pharmaceutical industry have a committee of six operating in Geneva whose sole job it is to infiltrate every international institution to prevent mandatory legislation against the . . . activities of multinationals' (private communication from a Member of the European Parliament).

It is too early to evaluate the practical impact of the UN family's new medicines policy. The Director-General of WHO stated in a report in 1978 (A32/2, p. 5) that in spite of the activities following the Colombo resolution 'an optimally co-ordinated drive is not taking place'. Two concrete projects are being implemented: the creation of a Caribbean Centre for Pharmaceuticals which will serve 'as a focal point for regional activities in the pharmaceutical sector and . . . undertake a set of functions, including central procurement, providing industrial co-operation, quality control, dissemination of information and training' (by UNDP and UNCTAD) and the setting up of a Pharmaceutical Centre in Africa for the 'transfer of technology to a group of countries for the production of simple drugs for local needs' (ID/204 p. 39) and as a demonstration and training centre (by UNIDO).

In UN policy statements emphasis is laid again and again on the request that the provision of medicines must be based on real health needs. In developing countries the assessment of these needs is fraught with difficulties. Data which in developed countries might serve as a basis for estimates, e.g. present consumption, prescribing patterns, disease prevalence and other epidemiological data, local production, imports, etc., may not be available. Where they are available they may not be good indicators, since in many developing countries only a small, often unrepresentative part of the population has access to medical care; also research and record-keeping methodology necessary for good reporting may be absent. It is therefore essential that assessment methods and the significance of available data be scrutinised very carefully. The reports so far appear to contain very little data or concrete advice in this area. With poor data or insufficient awareness of data quality, mistakes in policy may easily arise.

The discrepancy between the enunciation of criteria on which a policy claims to be based and concrete indications on how such criteria can in practice be applied leaves the observer sceptical. It is certainly welcome that WHO and other UN agencies no longer see medicines policy as a series of more or less isolated 'technical' problems but in its economic and social context; and a rational medicines policy of course should be based on real health needs, but as long as the change in policy is not translated into concrete operations nobody in real need will gain from it. Efforts are being made: the list of essential drugs should be of real help for many countries as a guideline for setting priorities, but in that area as in others some questions remain unanswered: why did UNIDO – an organisation concerned with industrialisation – work out a list of essential drugs quite a while before WHO started on its own? And why was neither that list nor the report of the relevant working group ever published? Why were we told by the UNCTAD information service that contrary to all reports UNCTAD is no longer involved in pharmaceuticals, nor in the work arising from the Colombo resolution? (This may of course just mean that UNCTAD has a badly informed information officer, but the result is the same: a discrepancy between facts and reports to the public.) The secrecy and evasiveness of the international bureaucracy, described and criticised by Bruun, Pan and Rexed (1975), appears to be unchanged.

The European Community

Among governmental international organisations the European Community is in a special situation, for it can legislate directly for its member states without the possibility for members to make major reservations once a text has been adopted by the governing body, the Council of Ministers. The EEC legislates through regulations which are directly applicable in all member countries and supersede national legislation, or through directives which aim at the approximation or harmonisation of national legislations; directives are binding, they state goals or standards, whereas the practical provisions on how to implement them are left to national legislation. The second characteristic to bear in mind is that the aim of these texts is primarily the elimination of barriers to trade within the Community, such as diverging or conflicting rules on production, standards and sale of goods. Any other policy emerging from Community legislation – at least in the areas ruled by directives – is therefore in some ways a by-product. Thus medicines policy in the EEC arises not primarily from health or social considerations, but as a result of the harmonisation of policies in member states necessary for the liberalisation of trade within the Community.

The field of pharmaceuticals has for some time been an area in which national governments in Europe have exercised controls in the service of public health. These controls are divergent and it is therefore a field in which a good deal of harmonisation is necessary before free trade in medicines becomes possible. Attempts at harmonisation started relatively early: a first directive 'on the approximation of provisions laid down by law, regulation or administrative action relating to proprietary medicinal products' was adopted in January 1965 (65/65/EEC). It applies to proprietary medicinal products defined as 'ready-prepared medicinal products marketed under a special name and in a special pack' for human use (Art. 1). Medicinal products are defined as substances or combinations of substances presented for treating or preventing disease or administered with a view to making a medical diagnosis or to restoring, correcting or modifying physiological functions (Art. 1). The directive states that no such product may be placed on the market without an authorisation by the competent authority of the particular member state. The authorisations shall be valid for five years and be renewable for further five-year periods on application by the holder. In order to obtain the authorisation the applicant has to submit:

qualitative and quantitative particulars of all the constituents of
the product;
a 'brief description of the method of preparation';
'therapeutic indications, contra-indications and side-effects';
'posology, pharmaceutical form, method and route of administration
and expected shelf life if less than three years';
'control methods employed by the manufacturer';
'results of: physico-chemical, biological or microbiological tests;
pharmacological and toxicological tests; clinical trials';
proof that the manufacturer is authorised in his own country to
produce proprietary products;
authorisations obtained in other countries to market the relevant
product.

In certain cases a list of published references may be substituted for
the test results of pharmacological and toxicological tests and clinical
trials. Authorisations shall be refused if, after verification of the
submitted documents and informations, 'it proves that the proprietary
medicinal product is harmful in the normal conditions of use, or that
its therapeutic efficacy is lacking or is insufficiently substantiated by
the applicant, or that its qualitative or quantitative composition is not
as declared' (Art. 5). Authorisations shall be suspended or revoked
'where the product proves to be harmful in the normal conditions of
use, or where its therapeutic efficacy is lacking, or where its qualitative
and quantitative composition is not as declared. Therapeutic efficacy
is lacking when it is established that therapeutic results cannot be
obtained with the proprietary product'.

The labelling requirements are designed to facilitate control: they
contain a series of numbers and names, but apart from the name of
the product and the active ingredients the only compulsory information
which might interest the consumer or the prescriber is the method of
administration. The directive is silent on dosage, indications, contraindications and side effects; nor is anything set forth in law about
package inserts.

Art. 24 states that within five years the directive shall be
progressively applied to products sold under previous authorisations.

The text is general and leaves a good many questions open, e.g.
what does harmful mean? What tests have to be carried out for the
results to be acceptable, etc.? It was, however, only a first step:
in May 1975 two further directives were adopted and filled some
of the more obvious gaps in the previous one. Directive 75/318/EEC

says that 'standards and protocols for the performance of tests and trials (. . .) are an effective means of control (. . .) and hence of protecting public health and can facilitate the movement of these products by laying down uniform rules'. It contains a long annex with detailed descriptions and definitions of concepts, quality control at various stages of manufacturing, toxicological and pharmacological tests and clinical trials. It also states that the concepts of harmfulness and therapeutic efficacy 'can only be examined in relation to each other and have only a relative significance depending on the progress of scientific knowledge and the use for which the (. . .) product is intended'.

Directive 75/319/EEC, known as the second directive, specifies how applications have to be drawn up and who is qualified to do it, how they are to be examined, what information the package insert (which is not compulsory although member states may require it) must contain. It also sets up a Committee for Proprietary Medicinal Products responsible for giving an opinion as to whether a particular product complies with the requirements set out in directive 65/65/EEC. The directive also provides for a new procedure for products to be marketed in several member countries: if an authorisation is granted in one country the applicant can request that the relevant dossier be forwarded to the Committee for Proprietary Medicinal Products and other member states provided that the request names at least five other countries. This forwarding is considered equivalent to the submission of an application in these countries and if no objection is raised within 120 days the product can be marketed in these states. If objections are raised, the Committee has to give an opinion. But since the authorisations remain national, conflicts between countries, i.e. if some nations grant and others refuse marketing authorisation, can only be solved by negotiation or, ultimately, by the European Court of Justice. By the end of 1978 the Committee had received only two applications under this new procedure and it was consulted by member states on only about 20 medicines.

A Council decision, also adopted in May 1975 (75/320/EEC) sets up a Pharmaceutical Committee. The preamble of the decision says: 'the implementation of the measures adopted by the Council as regards the approximation of the laws relating to proprietary medicinal products for human use may raise problems which should be jointly examined' and Article 2 states that the Committee shall examine any question relating to the application of directives and any other question in the field of proprietary medicinal products. The EEC Commission has to consult the Committee when preparing proposals for directives in the field of proprietary drugs. The Committee consists of 'senior experts in public health matters from the Member States' administrations' (Art. 3) and is chaired by a representative of the Commission.

The Committee is concerned with two areas: firstly questions arising directly from the application of the directives, e.g. the mutual information of competent authorities (75/319, Art. 30), legislation concerning older products (the second directive grants a period of 15 years for the progressive application to products placed on the market under previous provisions), the legal status of the 'scientific explanatory notes' for manufacturers and national authorities which are being worked out by the Committee for Proprietary Medicinal Products to specify the provisions of the annex of Directive 75/318. Secondly, it deals with more general matters of policy, e.g. is there a need for a directive about vaccines and sera which are excluded from the present ones? Should the explanatory notes lead to a new directive, etc.? The setting up of the Pharmaceutical Committee seems to be a first step towards a more purposeful shaping of a medicines policy in the Community. The Committee, however, has only a consultative status.

This series of directives and decisions makes the rules first laid down in 1965 more concrete and precise, but it does not guarantee that tests and experiments carried out in different countries and decisions taken by national authorities be uniform. But the 1975 measures were obviously seen as just a further step: Article 15 of the second directive says: 'in the light of experience the Commission shall, not later than four years after entry into force of this Directive, submit to the Council a proposal containing appropriate measures leading towards abolition of any remaining barriers to the free movement of proprietary medicinal products'. According to the head of the competent division in the Commission it is unlikely that a further directive would create a centralised European authorisation; a more likely procedure would be to negotiate a mutual recognition of national authorisations.

Since the 1975 texts *de facto* only came into force at the beginning of 1978 when the Federal Republic of Germany changed its drug legislation, it is difficult to assess their practical effect. Price differences for identical products in different EEC countries are considerable, as a report of the European Bureau of Consumer Unions (Consumers and the Cost of Pharmaceutical Products, BEUC, 1978) has documented. That report prompted the setting up of a working group on pharmaceutical prices meeting for the first time in May 1979. Trade mark protection remains strong: the European Court of Justice ruled in May 1978 that Hofmann La Roche had the right to oppose the sale of Valium Roche in Germany by the firm Centrafarm which had bought the product in England, where it was cheaper than the same product sold in Germany, repackaged it and sold it in Germany under the trade mark Valium Roche with the indication 'marketed by Centrafarm'. Free competition, which is supposed to be prompted by harmonisation and which in theory benefits the consumer, does not appear to be thriving. So far the statistics show no significant increase in intra-Community trade in medicines compared with imports and exports from and to third countries (see Table 8.5, p. 237). This is hardly surprising: the fact that Denmark has only two to three thousand medical specialities on the market whereas the UK and Germany have over 15,000 indicates strong differences in authorisation procedures and their underlying policies. It is likely to take a long time and a lot of political will to harmonise such policies effectively.

Up to now Community legislation on drugs concentrated on the conditions under which a product can be brought on the market. Efforts to widen this approach have not been very successful: a draft directive on publicity which was submitted to the Council of Ministers in 1967 was never discussed and eventually withdrawn. A new text is being prepared now, more stringent than the previous one, particularly in that it contains a clause stating that the rules of the directive are only minimum rules, i.e. member states can apply stricter controls. The draft as it was in 1979 (and it may still be amended by the Commission before submission to the European Parliament, the Economic and Social Council and eventually the Council) bans publicity to the general public for prescription drugs and for drugs relating to a list of some 50 diseases, prohibits the offer or promise to prescribers of gifts or other material benefits 'which are not of negligible value', restricts the distribution of samples to recipients who have requested them in writing and to quantities necessary for clinical appraisal of the product, and lays down what information has to be contained in any publicity material.[9] It requires control of advertising by member states without, however, specifying whether this control should be carried out *a priori* or *a posteriori*.

EEC representatives — like those of other organisations —

are reluctant to discuss how the Commission consults or co-operates with the pharmaceutical industry. Whereas there is now a consultative committee for consumers to which the Commission submitted the draft directive on publicity, there is no such formal way of consulting the industry. When regulations or directives are drafted the industries concerned often approach the relevant directorate. The pharmaceutical industry established an International Group of Pharmaceutical Industries of the EEC Countries (known under its French initials GIIP) in Brussels for this purpose. The Commission can also appoint industry representatives to the technical committees working on the drafts. Since the Commission refuses to disclose the composition of these committees, one is unable to confirm or refute the statement of Mr Edwards in the European Parliament in February 1979 that most of these committees are manned by representatives of the multinational companies.

The Commission intends to introduce legislation bearing on provision of information to prescribers. Apart from that there are so far no indications that future legislation will be based on wider considerations than the ones pertaining to the liberalisation of trade.

Conclusions

The UN system's policy has moved from simply trying to regulate international commerce of pharmaceuticals towards a more integrated medicines policy where the emphasis is laid firmly on economic and health needs of developing countries. Although it is too soon to expect the implementation of this policy to have led already to fundamental changes in member countries' medicines policy or provision systems, there are in the UN organisations discrepancies between claimed activities and actual operations which leave the observer somewhat sceptical.[10] And although real health needs are the linchpin of the UN agencies' medicines policy, there are so far no detailed concrete indications as to how such needs are to be assessed. One difficulty for the outside investigator is the fact that the UN organisations' methods of record keeping, library accessibility, bureaucratic and communication procedures are such that they often deny information about the internal workings of these organisations. It is a happy circumstance that such problems arise far less often at WHO where document catalogues are adequate and accessible and librarians eager to help.

It is strongly evident that there are divisive interests at work on or within the UN system, although because of the inaccessibility of information it is impossible to assess the weight of the various influences. The pharmaceutical industry is one profit-oriented and still influential force. The voting power of the Third World countries which accounts for the current position of the UN agencies is countered by the less visibly operating interests of the technologically advanced nations.

Apparent too is a lack of co-ordination within the group of UN organisations. Whereas WHO has no competence in areas relating to production, costs, transfer of technology, etc., UNCTAD, UNIDO and other agencies have no officially recognised competence in medicine and health (this is – we presume – demonstrated by the lack of publication or follow-up to UNIDO's list of essential drugs). Given on the one hand the comprehensive and interdisciplinary approach of the policies recommended by these agencies and, on the other hand, their limited areas of activities and competence, there can be no concrete implementation of such policies without a very close interagency co-ordination and co-operation. As far as co-operation is mentioned in reports, it appears to a large extent to be limited to informal and personal contacts at secretariat level.

Inside the agencies certain management practices serve perhaps less the task performance of mandated activities than the protection of bureaucrats from attacks which are so easily generated in a system composed of divisive national and economic interests. The best summary of this state of affairs is to be found in the book by Bruun, Pan and Rexed (1975) and its sequel Pan and Bruun (1979).

In contrast to the UN agencies, regional bodies have a more restricted focus. The functionally most developed regional unit, the EEC, is primarily a trade-stimulating entity. But however homogeneous its commercial value system, it is almost impossible to study its internal decision processes because these are not a matter for public record.

For the consumer, the external observer or the management expert it is readily seen that one of the immediate short-term needs – if there is to be improvement in the international co-ordination in the provision of medicines – is in the information systems, i.e. the organisations themselves.

Table 8.5: EEC Trade in Medicaments Pre-packaged for Retail Sale
Percentage of Intra-community Trade in Total Trade

	Imports	Exports
1974	81%	32%
1975	80%	31%
1976	79%	32%
1977	80%	31%
1978	79%	35%

Source: Official statistics, Statistics Office of the European Community.

Notes

I would like to thank Bror Rexed for his encouraging comments and Richard Blum, Kettil Bruun, Lynn Pan and Paschal Preston for their great patience and constructive advice.

1. Argentina, Australia, Austria, Bahrain, Barbados, Canada, Chile, Cyprus, Czechoslovakia, Denmark, Finland, France, Hungary, Israel, Italy, Madagascar, Malta, Netherlands, Poland, Portugal, Republic of Korea, Romania, Singapore, Spain, Sweden, Thailand, UK, USA, USSR.

2. Argentina, Australia, Belgium, Cyprus, Egypt, Finland, France, Iceland, Italy, Japan, Jordan, Mauritius, New Zealand, Norway, Poland, Portugal, Republic of Korea, Romania, Senegal, Spain, Sweden, Syrian Arab Republic, United Arab Emirates, United Kingdom, United States.

3. Scientific Group on Principles for Pre-clinical Testing of Drug Safety, TR 341. Scientific Group on Principles for the Clinical Evaluation of Drugs, TR 403. Clinical Pharmacology, TR 446. Principles for the Testing and Evaluation of Drugs for Carcinogenicity, TR 426. Evaluation and Testing of Drugs for Mutagenicity, TR 482. International Drug Monitoring: The Role of National Centres, TR 498, etc.

4. Biology and Pharmacology, later renamed Pharmacology and Toxicology and eventually Prophylactic, Diagnostic and Therapeutic Substances.

5. Lall (1978) quotes a total sales figure for the 34 leading firms of $18,134,500,000 for 1974 and states that promotional expenditure represents 15-25 per cent of sales. According to the UN Report 'Transnational Corporations and the Pharmaceutical Industry' (1979), the proportion spent on promotion is 20 per cent; in 1977 the amount spent in the US alone amounted to $1.9 billion dollars, based on total human dosage ethical drug sales (p. 47).

6. Required information includes: full designation of active ingredients, action and uses, dosage, form of administration, side effects, adverse reactions, precautions and contraindications, treatment in case of poisoning and references to literature.

7. We were unable to obtain a copy of this list or indeed any record of the meeting. We can therefore only wonder why a UNIDO meeting prepared such a list and why it was never published. The WHO list was published in 1977.

8. All the reports mention UNCTAD as a member of this task force. This is in contradiction with a statement of a representative of UNCTAD's Information Service who declared firmly that UNCTAD is no longer active in this field.

9. Qualitative and quantitative particulars of active ingredients, international and non-proprietary names; common name must be as legible as brand name;

therapeutic indications, contraindications, side effects and special precautions; directions for use of product (method of administration, duration of treatment if it should be limited, normal dosage), content of package and price.

10. On the basis of information obtained from the International Narcotics Control Board Pan and Bruun (1979) report that the statistics on psychotropic substances should be published by the autumn 1978. A report by the Board published in January 1979 refers to these statistics indicating the documents, reference number, but the document did not appear until the autumn of 1979.

References

Blum, R.H., Bovet, D. and Moore, J. (eds.) (1974). *Controlling Drugs: An International Handbook for Drug Classification*, San Francisco, Jossey-Bass

Bruun, K., Pan, K. and Rexed, I. (1975). *The Gentlemen's Club. International Control of Drugs and Alcohol*, University of Chicago Press

Bureau Européen des Unions de Consommateurs: Consumers and the Cost of Pharmaceutical Products. BEUC 1978

Djukanovic, V. and Mack, E.P. (1975). Alternative approaches to meeting basic health needs in developing countries. WHO

EEC (1978). The rules governing medicaments in the European Community. ISBN 92-825-0275-9

—— (1977/8). First Commission Report on the functioning of the Committee for Proprietary Medicinal Products and its impact on the development of intra-Community trade. Period 1977/78

—— (1978). Proceedings of the Court of Justice of the European Communities, Week 0 22 to 26 May

—— The Official Journal, the Official Statistics of the Statistics Office of the European Community and the Proceedings of the European Parliament were extensively used as sources.

Lall, S. (1978). The growth of the pharmaceutical industry in developing countries: problems and prospects. ID/204. United Nations Publication E.78.II.B.4

Pan, L. and Bruun, K. (1979). Recent developments in international drug control. *British Journal of Addiction 74* 141-60

UN (1979). Transnational corporations and the pharmaceutical industry. New York, 1979, ST/CTC/9

UNCTAD (1975). 5. Lall with UNCTAD secretariat: Major issues in Transfer of Technology to Developing Countries: A Case Study of the Pharmaceutical Industry. TD/B/C.6/4

—— (1977). Case studies in the transfer of technology: The pharmaceutical industry in India. TD/B/C.6/20

—— (1977). Case studies in the transfer of technology: Pharmaceutical policy in Sri Lanka. TD/B/C.6/21

—— Technology policy in the pharmaceutical sector in developing countries. UNCTAD/TT/7

UNICEF (1978). General Progress Report 1978, E/ICEF/658. A strategy for basic services. UNICEF

—— (1978). ECOSOC, Official Records 1978, supplement 14, E/1978/54, E/ICEF/655

UNIDO (1978). ID/14 Functions and activities of UNIDO

—— ID/162 Guide to Information Sources No. 20, Information sources on the pharmaceutical industry

—— ID/C15 Production Policy and its role in the development of

Pharmaceutical Industries in Developing Countries

—— (1969). ID/WG.37 Expert Working Group Meeting on the Establishment of Pharmaceuticals in Developing Countries, Budapest, May

—— (1977). Ex 24 First Panel Meeting of Industrial Experts on the Pharmaceutical Industry, Vienna

—— (1978). ID/WG.267 Second Panel of Experts on the Pharmaceutical Industry, Vienna, February

—— (1971). ID/WG.116 Expert Group Meeting on the Production and Distribution of Contraception in the Developing Countries, New York, November

—— (1978). ID/WG.271 Production of Drugs from medicinal plants in developing countries, Lucknow, March

—— (1979). ID/WG.292 Interregional meeting to prepare for Consultations on the Pharmaceutical Industry, Cairo, January

WHO Chronicle (1979). Science and Technology for Health Promotion in developing countries. WHO document for the UN Conference on Science and Technology for Development

WHO Official Records. Handbook of Resolutions and Decisions. Documents of the World Health Assembly. Summary records and documents of the Executive Board. International Digest of Health Legislation. Technical Report Series (abbreviated: TR)

9 COHERENT POLICIES ON DRUGS: FORMULATION AND IMPLEMENTATION

Wilfred Lionel and Andrew Herxheimer

9.1 The Need for a Policy and its Purpose

Drugs of proven efficacy and safety play an important role in the provision of adequate health care and have made possible the prevention and treatment of disease with significant reduction in morbidity and mortality. Unfortunately a good proportion of the drugs available are of little importance in terms of essential health care and are marketed mainly because they can be sold and not because they benefit the health of the population. A high proportion of the expenditure on drugs by governments and individuals is thus wasted on preparations which are of little value in terms of local health needs. The sums involved are large — of the order of 10 per cent of the total health budget in the developed countries and as much as 30-40 per cent in some developing countries.

There is therefore an urgent need to identify drugs that are important in terms of the health needs of a population and to ensure that they are of proved quality and available at reasonable cost to all who need them. Where appropriate, the local development and production of drugs needed for health care should be encouraged. To achieve these aims it is essential to formulate policies covering all aspects of drug development, manufacture, and use. They will involve health services and education as well as the industrial and trade sectors. Such drug policies are or should be an important part of the health programme of a country, whatever its social and economic development or political ideology.

9.2 Considerations in Formulating a Policy

For formulation of realistic drug policies it is necessary to have accurate information on the prevalence of treatable diseases and the drugs (which ones and in what quantities) available for providing health care, the technical and administrative personnel available to implement the policies, and the extent of financial resources. It is also necessary to know what are the practices and beliefs of those who consume medicines and what will constitute effective education to increase the wise use of medicines by individuals and families. Where such information is inadequate, studies should be carried out to obtain it. This requires people trained in epidemiology, demography, economics, and preventive, psychological and cultural medicine, as well as clinicians. Countries lacking such expertise can seek help from international organisations such as WHO.

9.3 Policy Areas

9.3.1 Registration and Licensing of Medicines

One of the most important aspects of State regulation is the registration and licensing of drugs. The primary purpose of registration is to ascertain all the medicines sold; that of licensing is to ensure that only effective and acceptably safe pharmaceuticals of good quality are marketed. Registration must precede the introduction of a system of licensing: the two are merely successive stages of the same process of control. Indeed the term registration is often applied to the whole process (IFPMA, 1980).

The regulatory authority should set out the information required in an application for registration and the conditions that must be fulfilled for a licence to be granted. Before the authority can decide whether to license a particular medicine it needs information of various kinds about it. This should include:

> details of manufacture;
> whether the preparation conforms to recognised pharmacopoeial standards;
> stability tests and their results;
> results of pharmacological and toxicological tests in animals and the methods used;
> results of bioavailability studies where necessary;
> results of studies in man, including controlled clinical trials;
> available information on adverse effects;
> copies of labels and package inserts which would be used on the products.

To assess the information submitted requires the setting up of a committee of experts to advise whether the data are sufficient for licensing and whether the application should be accepted or rejected.

In licensing drugs for marketing a definite policy must be adopted on the criteria used; whether to license all drugs conforming to the requirements of efficacy, safety and quality, or to consider other aspects as well. One recognises at this point that issues involving larger values enter into medicines policy. For example, a nation with a very limited health budget and serious health problems may be forced to develop treatment priorities. In such cases, if its application is to a minor ailment but the costs of drug importation by a state system are great, the state may decide to forgo the 'luxury' of the medicament. Such a decision runs contrary to the interest of an individual suffering from the ailment, and that suffering must then be considered a cost of the policy.

Another issue arises in countries where all equivalent products are not freely licensed. Thus a new drug may be refused a licence, even if the medicine is safe and effective, if an equivalent product already exists on the market at an equivalent or lower price. Such a decision may have the cost of (unintentionally) producing a monopoly to the existing sellers and will deprive the state and its taxpayers of any benefits from competitive price reductions. Such benefits are by no means assured, however, in free-market economies, insofar as cartel agreements — which may be made outside a country by international manufacturers (e.g. the 'Dolder Club') — may control pricing in market countries. A possible advantage of limited licensing for equivalent products is that better wholesale prices may be achieved by larger bulk purchases, be these by the state or private importers.

Countries without adequate trained personnel or other necessary facilities will have to base their decisions on registration on evaluations made in countries with such facilities where such data have been submitted. This in turn requires — as we shall propose — international facilities for the exchange of data on new drugs, and on regulatory decisions made (See Section 9.5 of this chapter).

Legislation should permit withdrawal of registration of the licensed product where new data invalidate an original submission on which the initial decision to register was based. It is best to limit the period of registration, so that regular review, say every 5 or 10 years, is built into the system.

A recent book edited by Wardell (1978) compares the licensing procedures in use in seven European countries, Canada and New Zealand. The effectiveness of the different procedures is, however, hard to judge from these descriptions.

9.3.2 Legal and Administrative Restrictions on Supply

For every medicine the regulatory authority must decide how freely it should be available.

If the medicine is needed for self-medication, then it should be available to the public without prescription. Some medicines, for example, aspirin or paracetamol tablets, may be appropriately sold in any kind of shop, though it is desirable to limit the quantity of these sold in a single purchase. The sale of others that carry some risk of abuse, for example, sedative antihistamines or cough suppressants, may be better restricted to drug stores and/or pharmacies. For certain medicines it may be made mandatory to record all sales in a register, so that abuse can be more readily detected.

If use of the medicine requires special skill or may be hazardous, then it is desirable to supply it only on the prescription of a health professional, usually a doctor. In some cases prescription by a midwife, nurse (eg. drugs used in childbirth, contraceptives) or other trained health worker is appropriate. The decision for a particular medicine will be influenced by the urgency of the need for it and by the accessibility and capabilities of the local primary health care workers. For example where malaria is endemic and health workers scarce, one or more antimalarial drugs must be freely available. In Europe, where malaria is uncommon and health services are easily accessible, it is reasonable to supply antimalarial drugs only on prescription. Again the distribution of an oral contraceptive by a village general store may be appropriate in a developing country, but unacceptable in a country with efficient and well-staffed family-planning and obstetric services. In the first setting the risks of an unwanted pregnancy are much greater than in the second. The benefit/risk ratio of oral contraception is consequently also much greater.

Drugs that are too dangerous or difficult to use without special experience and facilities – for example drugs used in cancer chemotherapy, or in the management of drug dependence – are best restricted to the appropriate specialists. Since relatively few specialists in a country will be affected it is simpler to control the supply of such drugs administratively, for example through hospitals recognised for the purpose, than by a regulation requiring a special type of prescription.

A change in the way in which a medicine is used or abused, or the identification of previously unrecognised hazards, may be reasons for changing the prescription status of a drug. For example, medicines containing phenacetin or clioquinol were sold without prescription for decades, but have recently been either banned or put on prescription in an increasing number of countries (Inman 1980).

9.3.3 Priority or Essential Drugs

Drugs which are considered essential for the health care of the people need to be identified, so that where financial resources are limited, the money at present spent on all drugs could be used primarily for those which serve essential health needs and therefore deserve priority.

Drugs which should be given priority would vary from country to country depending on the pattern of prevalent diseases, the type of health personnel available for health care and the financial resources. Other factors which may influence selection of these priority drugs are the stability of drugs and the availability of proper storage facilities, and also genetic and demographic factors.

Guidelines for selecting these priority drugs have been published by the World Health Organisation, together with a model list of essential drugs (WHO, 1977, 1979). They should be drugs of proved efficacy and acceptable safety that are needed for the prevention and treatment of the most prevalent diseases and which would give wide coverage to the health needs of the majority. The types of health workers available to diagnose illness and prescribe the drugs should be considered. A smaller range of drugs will be needed in primary health care than in hospitals. Cost is also an important selection criterion and cost effectiveness should be taken into account when considering the diseases which require treatment with drugs. The implementation of an essential drug policy would discourage the use of ineffective drugs and waste of money on them. Carol Barker and her colleagues (1978) give some interesting examples from Mozambique, which show well how such a policy can be applied in preparing a National Formulary.

Here again one recognises that the ordering of scarce resource allocations by health priorities on the part of state (or regional agencies deprives either a prescribing physician (or other healer) or the patient of there being available any — or perhaps only the optimal — medicament for a 'low priority' illness. Priorities when these are set officially are decided via several criteria, all of which must be explicitly and publicly debated. Does one exclude from treatment for reasons of drug import and associated health care costs rare diseases when they are fatal? Or common diseases fatal for populations considered expendable, e.g. the elderly, the addicted, the demented, or newborn in a nation with population control problems? Or does one, in a less fierce posture, simply exclude medicaments for illnesses judged minor? One asks of course, who makes that judgement: the patient? or the state? Such questions are further complicated by the relative inefficacy of many treatments. For example, many anti-cancer drugs, even when used in the best way, are effective in only a small proportion of cases, and those who will be helped can usually not be identified beforehand.

One sees the human and political implications of such regulatory control decisions and may shy away from them on the assumed grounds that free-market licensing policy assures the better world. Unfortunately that cannot be assured, for where health care resources are inadequate to finance the provision of medicines for all the ill, it is the case that, where no public care system exists, the uninsured poor will be untreated, no matter how severe their illness. And when medical care *is* provided by the state, as long as money is insufficient, the state capabilities will be limited so that some of the sick will still not receive the medicines they need. This problem is of course exaggerated insofar as a correlate of poverty is likely to be failure to seek — or to have readily accessible — medical services as such.

It is evident then that in the absence of a perfect world, some patients will not — no matter what economic value-system reigns — receive the medicines appropriate for their illnesses. The best an economic policy on medicine registration and importation can do is to be honest about its assumptions and criteria, constantly evaluate the real-life impact, costs and benefits of its policies, involve the affected citizenry (consumers and professionals) in the decision-making and seek a programme of preventive medicine, cheaper efficacious drugs, reduced waste of drugs that are available, and efficiency in medical/administrative programmes. Under such real demands, and with real human suffering the price of any decision, one may well argue that political/economic dogmas or ideology have no place in medicines policy. The requirements for policy are pragmatic, empirical, rational and humane. These are values, we believe, inherent in any decent professional committed to health care and medicines policies.

9.3.4 Licensing of Other Drugs in Use

In the case of traditional or herbal remedies which have been in use for centuries and are still enjoying widespread popularity among the people of a country it may be necessary to permit their use and marketing although their efficacy cannot be assessed. One distinguishes a number of levels of use of these folk medicines. There are those primarily considered as foods or beverages and which are locally produced or which grow in the wild. The only possible control over their use, which is in the hands of the family or patient, is by education should it be found that the local remedies are not safely used by the local population. Thus one continuing effort in pharmacognosy is the evaluation of local remedies to test for toxicity. When toxicity is discovered, and there is epidemiological evidence of ill effects from local customs, the educational as well as local medical apparatus must be put into gear.

At another level there exists a wide range of remedies (real or imagined) which are sold. At this point economic as well as health considerations emerge, for money spent on a packaged inefficacious folk remedy may exclude purchase of a useful medicine. But profit motives of retailers, folk healers and manufacturers enter into the picture, so that – as in the pharmaceutical industry – there is resistance to control. Again the policy commitment must be to drug evaluation and to control by education when toxicity is demonstrated, or when inefficacious 'remedies' are used to the exclusion of effective ones.

An urban medical practitioner may tend to overlook the vast use of folk remedies, not only in the peasant or tribal societies, but in technological ones as well. Also overlooked may be the importance of naturally occurring compounds, either in pharmacognosy as sources of discovery for very important manufactured synthesised medicines (consider aspirin, morphine, penicillin), but also as a source of potentially toxic effects (consider opium, betel nut, coca, psilocybin, ergot). The actual practices in use also remind us that drug policy decisions relate closely to issues involving the safety of foods, beverages and cosmetics.

9.3.5 Quality Control

As stated earlier, the production of drugs of good quality is a complex technological activity which can go wrong. Effective measures for controlling quality are therefore needed. This should not be left entirely to the individual manufacturers. It should be the task of the state to ensure that the drugs imported or manufactured locally are of good quality. This can be done by:

(1) Introducing legislation to ensure that drugs manufactured locally are produced using good manufacturing practices to meet established quality specifications as set out by organisations such as WHO.

(2) Carrying out quality control at all stages of manufacture and not limiting it to checks on samples of the finished products.
(3) Setting up analytical control laboratories to perform such quality control work either at national level or at a regional level to serve two or more neighbouring states.
(4) Training of personnel to perform quality control work in the laboratory as well as to inspect manufacturing records and premises.

9.3.6 Information and Education

Accurate and objective information on drugs must be available to help those prescribing drugs to make proper decisions in selecting the drugs and to learn how to use them to the best effect. Lack of knowledge or inaccurate or misleading information on drugs have led to their unnecessary or wrong use, with increase in costs both to the state as well as the patients. Surveys of prescribing habits in different countries have revealed this time and time again. Adverse reactions to drugs are often due to improper use or lack of awareness of their toxicity on the part of prescribing doctors and/or patients. Many adverse reactions could be prevented if prescribers were better informed about the drugs they use (George and Kingscombe, 1980).

Those who prescribe drugs must therefore have an adequate accurate knowledge of the properties of the drugs available for their use, not only to obtain the best results, but also to avoid doing harm with them. Excessive detail on drugs is not necessary but only that amount actually required for their judicious use. The information that must be provided should therefore be essentially practical. It should help the prescriber to get the best results with the minimum of harmful effects: to achieve the lowest risk/benefit ratio.

At present, the pharmaceutical industry plays a very important role in providing information on drugs to the medical profession and doctors have come to rely heavily on such information in the choice of a drug. Unfortunately the information from drug manufacturers is often biased toward the drugs they are promoting and often the interests of drug promotion are in conflict with the provision of unbiased information. This does not imply that all promotional literature is exaggerated or bad. In fact, part of the information provided is helpful, but there is no doubt that heavy promotion has to a great extent been responsible for excessive and irrational prescribing. But many prescribers have to rely on drug manufacturers for information because they often get very little from sources that are independent of the drug industry.

The function of providing information on drugs cannot therefore be left solely to pharmaceutical companies. It should be the responsibility of the health authorities to provide independent information. This has been done in some countries, for example Scandinavia and in developing countries such as Peru, where a compilation of monographs on basic drugs is published by the national authorities.

Unfortunately many of the developing countries do not have the expertise or the facilities to provide such information and it is here that international co-operation and organisations like the World Health Organisation can help. As far as essential drugs are concerned, a compact book in loose-leaf form or in the form of cards for storage and reference could be published by WHO. These would serve as a guide to individual countries in the production of similar material adapted to their local needs. In view of the rapid developments in knowledge about drugs, such information must regularly be updated. The information should provide in more or less summary form all that is necessary for their safe and effective use.

Regulations should be framed to control advertising and other promotion of drugs, and advertisements should be approved by the regulatory authorities to prevent exaggerated claims. Labelling and package inserts of drug packs for export and for domestic use should as a rule include the same clinical indications and warnings.

Education and training about drugs and their use are essential to ensure the rational use of drugs and their importance is increasingly recognised. Such education and training should begin in the undergraduate years of the medical curriculum or during the initial training period of other health workers who have to prescribe drugs. Emphasis should be laid on those aspects of pharmacology necessary for the rational use of drugs. Academic teaching on ideal drug therapy is of little value in most situations where the facilities to practise such therapy are limited. The students must be taught the use of drugs in a way which would yield optimum results in the context of the situation prevailing in the particular country, often under far from ideal conditions. The students must also be taught to discriminate between unbiased information on drugs and unsubstantiated promotional claims of the manufacturers. They must be taught the principles of clinical trials so that they can examine the evidence on which claims are made for drugs, and properly assess claims. Economy in prescribing is also an important aspect in the selection of an appropriate drug and unfortunately it is one aspect of drug therapy which is least stressed in undergraduate education. Such information serves to reduce unnecessary expenditure by helping in the identification and selection of cheaper therapeutic equivalents in place of expensive preparations.

There is also the problem of keeping abreast of the rapidly increasing knowledge on new as well as existing drugs, particularly knowledge about their practical use.

Unfortunately so far, in many countries very little continuing education has been attempted to enable practitioners to keep abreast of the essential ever-increasing knowledge about drugs required for rational prescribing. It is in the public interest to ensure continuing education on the value and safety of existing as well as new drugs so that standards of therapy may be maintained and even improved and the misuse of drugs minimised. This is discussed in detail in Chapter 5.

There is evidence that continuing professional education – where it is available – is pursued only by a minority of practitioners. In response some countries require attendance at coursework or impose requalifying examinations as a condition for the renewal of physicians' licences. There can be strong resistance to the demand for a continued demonstration of professional responsibility and competence, but any commitment to high standards of care requires such conditional licensing of which demonstrated knowledge in current therapeutics must be a part.

Governments are also wise to publish or sponsor regular publication of a bulletin on drugs, with the help of experts available in the country. Such bulletins are now published in many countries, e.g. in the USA, the Netherlands, the UK and Australia. In some countries non-governmental organisations also publish bulletins, for example the *Medical Letter* in the US, *Drug and Therapeutics Bulletin* in the UK, *Arzneimittelbrief* and *Arzneitelegramm* in the Federal Republic of Germany. Regular refresher courses planned and designed to meet the needs of prescribers as well as the content of drug bulletins, should be controlled by professional bodies, not by the pharmaceutical industry, though the latter may have useful contributions to make (Medico-Pharmaceutical Forum, 1978). Where people who can carry out such activities are lacking, the World Health Organisation could be asked to help by providing the necessary facilities and experts to design and start such courses in the context of the needs of the particular country.

The current arrangements in several European countries and in New Zealand for providing independent drug information and continuing education for doctors are outlined in Wardell's book (1978).

9.3.7 Surveillance of Drug Utilisation

It is well known that the drugs which are available are not always used in the correct way for the correct indications. Therefore while it is important to provide prescribers with continuing information on drug efficacy and safety, it is also necessary to assess the effects of giving them such information. Regular surveillance of utilisation patterns of the essential drugs in a country will help to determine the extent of inappropriate, excessive or insufficient utilisation of drugs. The results will enable decisions to be taken in instituting corrective measures to promote rational prescribing. In this way health care can be improved and unnecessary expenditure on drugs reduced or eliminated. Drug utilisation can be studied at various levels. Studies of the gross sales figures in terms of quantities of drugs obtained from local drug manufacturers or importers (or the state drug agency where the state is the sole importer) will give information on what drugs are used, changes in the drugs used over a given period and the extent of use of different drugs or classes of drugs. They can also give a rough measure of the effects on prescribing habits of providing unbiased information on drugs.

Surveys of prescriptions, made with the collaboration of prescribers as well as pharmacists, will give an idea again of the drugs prescribed, the indications for which they have been used and in which diseases, the dosage, and the total amounts prescribed together with the age and sex of the patients for whom the drugs have been prescribed. Similar information about the use of drugs could also be obtained from the hospital records. Such studies may help to identify causes of over-consumption of drugs such as the prescribing of excessive quantities of drugs to individuals, excessive frequency of prescription for certain drugs, use of inappropriate drugs for a particular clinical indication and unnecessary prescribing of two or more drugs when one would suffice.

Field surveys on the extent of drug usage in a selected population would show to what extent people are taking prescribed drugs as instructed (compliance), and self-prescribed (non-prescription) drugs. More intensive observational research can refine survey data, including identification of patient and illness characteristics most associated with unwise use of medicines.

Analysis of the data from all such utilisation studies together with health survey data on the prevalence of different diseases in a country can show up not only overconsumption of drugs but also under-utilisation. For example, comparison of the data on the extent of use of antihypertensive drugs with the prevalence of hypertension in a particular country may reveal underutilisation of antihypertensive drugs. Further study would be required to discover the reasons for this and to suggest possible ways of improving utilisation.

In this connection, it is highly desirable to use standardised methods for studies of drug utilisation because this enables data from different countries to be compared. Such comparisons have been made between some European countries (Symposium, 1976).

The minimal incidence of adverse reactions to drugs in relation to the extent of their use, i.e. the apparent risk, can also be estimated from drug utilisation studies. In addition they can help in evaluating the effectiveness of warnings about serious reactions to particular drugs.

Every country should establish a scheme for performing drug utilisation studies. Where trained personnel are not available the World Health Organisation should assist such states in undertaking and evaluating the results of such studies.

9.3.8 Safety of Medicines and Drug Monitoring

All drugs may produce more or less serious adverse effects in some people and in some circumstances. Although numerous animal toxicology tests are done before a drug is marketed, many of these adverse effects do not come to light till it is used clinically.

Serious reactions are difficult to detect because they are rare and they may be recognised only after the drug has been in use for several years. Often a cause-and-effect relationship is not easy to establish as many of the reactions are non-specific in character. Also adverse reactions are often not reported, or reports if available are scattered in the literature.

Methods are therefore needed to detect such adverse effects at the earliest possible moment so that prompt warning can be given to users and if necessary the use of the drug restricted or even withdrawn.

For this purpose a national adverse reaction monitoring centre is essential and it should provide facilities for spontaneous reporting of adverse effects both from hospitals and from general practice. The monitoring centre should have the personnel to collect and analyse reports and communicate any important information to doctors. Such a centre should also be able to provide advice about adverse reactions.

Since the pre-clinical and clinical studies before marketing cannot reveal the complete potential toxicity of a drug, particularly with long-term use, it is useful to have some follow-up of the safety and efficacy of a new drug for a period of time after marketing. Such 'post-marketing surveillance' or 'monitored release' should be carried out by regulatory authorities who would require feedback of information from the limited number of prescribers allowed use of the drug. Such a method is useful where the safety of a drug for long-term use has to be determined. Monitored release of new drugs would give a more accurate picture of their safety from long-continued general use – information which cannot be obtained in pre-registration trials limited to a few hundred patients given the drug for short periods. Drug monitoring is very fully discussed in two recent books edited by Gross and Inman (1977) and Inman (1980).

9.3.9 Local Production

Countries differ widely in their capacity to manufacture pharmaceutical products. They fall into four groups:

(1) those with no pharmaceutical industry;
(2) those where some packaging and formulation is carried out;
(3) those where a substantial number of essential drugs is formulated locally;
(4) those producing their own drugs from raw materials and basic chemicals.

It is widely recognised that health regions as well as individual nations will benefit from increased competence in the production of drugs needed locally. The degree of commitment to production and research will depend on regional and local economic capacities and personnel resources as well as on the discrepancies between existing medicines provision and actual need. The advantages of such developments are:

(a) self-sufficiency in at least the essential drugs and less dependence on foreign supplies;
(b) more reliable supply which can be adapted to changing needs and therefore less risk of shortages;
(c) saving on foreign exchange in some circumstances;
(d) provision of local employment.

However, some nations have called for independent and national self-sufficiency for essential drug production. Such national proposals are by no means universally endorsed.

The only disadvantage to be set against these is that small-scale production may be uneconomical and more expensive than importation of the finished product.

The setting up of pharmaceutical manufacturing units is not a simple task, for sophisticated techniques have to be employed if the standards set up by the developed countries are to be met. This presents a serious problem for developing countries. Therefore international or regional assistance to develop and expand local pharmaceutical manufacture will often be needed. UNIDO, the United Nations Industrial Development Organisation, has considerable experience of helping countries to set up pharmaceutical manufacture (UNIDO, 1978).

It is evident that economic benefits accrue when production and marketing enjoy rational specialisation and 'economies of scale', i.e. it is usually cheaper to produce – or buy– in bulk. Thus nations establishing their own industries under conditions where neither natural resources, manufactured chemical components or skilled labour are more cheaply available do necessarily incur higher costs than production centres enjoying these advantages. These higher costs can be offset by freight costs, import taxation (an arbitrary imposition and certainly not one applied to state importations), or international cartel pricing.

Thus, when self-sufficiency is argued for, there can be undue costs to emerging nations in establishing local industries where resources or demand cannot support them. While restrictive trade practices may enable such an industry to survive, that survival becomes inevitably a tax on local consumers, the tax being the difference between the price of cheaper imported products and the higher local production costs subsidised by the state – or by prices paid by consumers. While the best examples of such costly local industries are to be seen flying through the air (the subsidised flag airlines), a local pharmaceutical industry can prove to be quite costly as well.

While national self-sufficiency itself can be a costly avenue to development, regional co-operation or other international arrangements may provide a much more beneficial set of outcomes and are to be strongly recommended, in harmony with UNCTAD proposals.

Gish and Feller (1979) provide a more detailed discussion of the issues involved in pharmaceutical production in developing countries.

9.3.10 Drug Exports

Government control of drug exports should also be an essential part of the drug policy as this would greatly help countries without trained people or facilities to test the efficacy and quality of imported drugs. The governments of most countries tend to regard any export as desirable and therefore to encourage such exports whatever the quality of the drug exported. In the case of drugs the exporting country has a responsibility to ensure that only therapeutically useful good-quality drugs are sent to other countries. The principle of caveat emptor seems particularly inappropriate when the importing country has little or no way of testing the drugs. However, it is too much to expect the drug regulatory authority of an exporting country to decide on the indications and warnings that would be appropriate to various importing countries. A reasonable compromise would be for the authority to inform its counterpart in the importing country whether the product is licensed, and if so what restrictions there are on its sale. If it is not licensed because it is produced only for export, then the authority should state whether an application for a product licence would be granted, and whether the manufacturer's plant and procedures had passed the official inspection.

9.3.11 Procurement of Drugs not Produced Locally

Since pharmaceuticals are among the most needed products for a country, there must be an efficient procurement system in each country. Depending on the policy of the government this can be a State monopoly or make use of both government and private importers. Whatever the method of procurement, systematic enquiries (see preceding section) or investigations must be made to determine the status of the manufacturers and their manufacturing practices, the reliability of quality assurance provided, and the registration status in the country of origin. Wherever necessary, bioavailability and therapeutic equivalence must be considered. Gish and Feller (1979) consider drug procurement in detail.

9.3.12 Drug Distribution

An efficient distribution system is required to ensure that drugs are promptly and easily available to those who need them. Any breakdown in the distribution system will interfere with the delivery of health care.

In many countries distribution of drugs is a function of both the state and the private sector. A government organisation may exist to

procure and distribute pharmaceuticals. Supplies to the private sector
are made by private importers or wholesalers who obtain supplies from
the private importer and in some instances from the state as well.
In some countries the state is the sole importer and distributor. The
choice of the distribution system is a matter of government policy,
but whether it is publicly or privately owned it should be efficient
so that drugs are available wherever they are needed. The organisation
of a distribution system should include adequate storage facilities,
proper inventory control and good transport facilities and maintenance services. The problems of distribution in Third-World countries
are examined more fully by Gish and Feller (1979).

9.3.13 Payment for Medicines

In every system of health care it must be decided how medicines
are to be paid for. At one extreme the health-care budget bears the
whole cost of all medicines, at the other the individual consumer
pays the full price of any medicine he needs when he does so. The
disadvantages of these extreme policies are obvious. To provide
medicines 'free' (in fact of course out of taxes or insurance
contributions) encourages wasteful prescribing and excessive demands
from patients. On the other hand, many who are poor or not working
cannot afford to pay for medicines. For these reasons most governmental and private health services impose some limits on the free
supply of medicines. These limits are of two kinds:

(1) Free supplies are restricted to certain categories of person,
e.g. dependent children, pregnant women, pensioners, those in
receipt of social security benefits.
(2) Free (or low-cost) supplies are restricted to certain categories
of drugs.

In the British National Health Service, persons who are not in an
exempt category such as those mentioned, have to pay a prescription
charge of £1 for every item. For the majority of medicines, though
not for all, this is less than the price a pharmacist would charge for a
private prescription. Exceptions are made for hospital inpatients,
who get all drugs free, patients treated for a sexually transmitted
disease in special clinics, and patients with certain life-long endocrine
deficiencies, such as myxoedema. No prescription charge is levied
for contraceptive preparations, since the state can save large sums
through their use; abortions and unwanted children cost very much

more. Products that are advertised directly to the public may not be prescribed in the Health Service. Apart from these, so-called border-line substances, which are mainly foods and toilet preparations with some limited medicinal uses, can be prescribed only for specified medicinal uses, otherwise the patient has to pay the full cost. These preparations are listed in MIMS (Monthly Index of Medical Specialities), a commercial compendium.

A limited list of medicines (Pharmaceutical Benefits) that may be prescribed is operated, for example in Australia (1979), New Zealand and Sweden. Preparations that are not listed, or quantities greater than those permitted have to be paid for by the patient.

Many countries have reimbursement schemes, in which the patient pays the full cost, or a high proportion of the cost of his medicine, and then can claim back some or all of this amount. Such schemes can become quite complex and expensive, as in France.

The simpler the rules that determine who has to pay how much, the less the cost of administration. But simple rules are perhaps more liable to cause inequitable anomalies and hardship. A limited list of drugs can help doctors to prescribe more rationally, and to resist overly demanding patients as well as promotional pressure from manufacturers. However, manufacturers in a drug-exporting country may justly fear that if their product is not on the pharmaceutical benefits or 'reimbursed' list in their home country, then it will be rejected by the authorities in importing countries. The arguments for and against limited prescribing lists continue to be hotly debated. In the UK the Department of Health is firmly against it (Deitch 1980). In France the complex Social Security regulations concerning reimbursement have caused increasing problems. In 1979 the Minister of Health commissioned a special inquiry into the causes of waste of medicines and possible remedies. The report (Arbon *et al.* 1979) concluded that the reimbursement procedures were certainly contributing to the inappropriate use of medicines, though other factors seemed to be more important.

9.4 The Formulation and Implementation of Policies

9.4.1 Advice and Decisions

National policies relating to medicines have important political implications, and responsibility must rest with a minister, usually the Minister of Health. He will need detailed advice from individuals who are competent and experienced in clinical medicine, pharmacology, toxicology, pharmacy, pharmaceutical manufacture, economics and civil service procedures and administration. Some of these experts will work full-time as civil servants in the ministry, others may act as part-time paid or unpaid advisers while continuing their professional work, for example in the practice and teaching of medicine, of pharmacology or of pharmacy.

9.4.2 Organisation

The parts of a ministry of health and ministries that deal with medicines can be organised in a variety of ways. The reasons for the variety are mainly historical: the organisations have grown piecemeal in response to changing and variously perceived needs. Often only those aspects of policy that directly concern health are managed in the ministry of health.

Other aspects may be dealt with in other ministries, for example, matters concerning the development and operation of the pharmaceutical industry may come under the ministry of industry, the training of doctors and pharmacists under the ministry of education, the prices of medicines sold to the public under a department of prices and consumer protection, the control of addictive drugs under a ministry of the interior or justice. Ideally it might be best to locate all these activities in the ministry of health, but if this is not practicable then at least that ministry should be responsible for health-related coordination and advice. Whether or not all the functions relating to medicines are performed in one ministry or in several, it is necessary to organise the business dealt with. Distinct areas that may need to be managed by separate units or subunits in the civil services are:

(1) licensing of drugs and of manufacturers;
(2) adverse reaction monitoring, post-marketing surveillance;
(3) standards for drugs and quality control;
(4) assessment of pharmaceutical needs, purchase, supply, distribution;
(5) information and education about medicines, monitoring of prescribing patterns;
(6) prevention of misuse of drugs;
(7) manpower needs, training, employment in pharmacy, pharmacology, clinical pharmacology, and in the pharmaceutical industry;
(8) the determination of needs and priorities in therapeutic research,

and the commissioning of important research projects;
(9) the development and sustenance of a healthy pharmaceutical
industry; exports of medicines.

Policies in these diverse areas cannot be adequately formulated and
implemented without expert advice from outside the civil service.
The particular experts who are consulted must be among the leaders
in their field, respected by their colleagues and in touch with them.
Often their advice will be given informally to the minister and his
civil servants, but formality is more appropriate when the advice is
to be published. It can then help to stimulate public discussion of
a proposed policy, or to make a ministerial decision better understood
by and acceptable to those affected by it. Where formal outside advice
is regularly needed it is useful to give the advisers official status. In
many countries the committees and commissions that advise on the
licensing of medicines, or on reimbursement schemes, are established
by law and the names of the members are published. In the UK for
example, the Medicines Commission and the Committee on Safety
of Medicines are statutory bodies set up under the provisions of
the Medicines Act (1968), to advise the Health Ministers on defined
matters (Medicines Commission, etc., Annual Reports). These
bodies are independent in mind – they are not the creatures of
the minister, but totally dependent on the minister's civil servants
for secretarial and administrative services.

The nature of the working relationship between the chairman
and the civil servants who do the background work for such a
committee determines whether there is a clear separation between
'outside' views and the 'departmental' view, or whether the
distinction tends to be blurred. Technically the committee advises
the minister on the matters put before it by the civil servants,
and the 'licensing authority', that is the civil servants on behalf
of the minister, make the decision, for example to grant a licence.
The authority is not legally bound to accept the advice, but merely
to seek it. However, in practice the advice is almost always accepted.
Presented here is, in essence, the European model. In North America,
the chief of the agency is responsible and not the Departmental
Secretarial head.

The minister remains responsible for all decisions, but he and
his servants can nevertheless shelter behind the advice of the outside
experts. This arrangement offers all concerned some protection
against real or apparent arbitrariness or injustice. To assure that a

'public' consciousness is inherent in all such governmental and
advisory activities, a ministry may well wish a respected consumer
or public-interest organisation to nominate private citizens to sit as
members of decision-making groups. Naturally, all proceedings
affecting policy must yield records that can be inspected by the
media or interested parties.

9.4.3 Laws and Regulations

Laws and regulations are needed where it is considered important
to ensure the observance of certain standards of behaviour by
individuals and by corporate bodies. This is the case for the
manufacture, sale, advertising, prescribing and dispensing of medicines.
The laws and regulations must specify the standards required, and the
categories of persons to be permitted to manufacture, sell, prescribe
or dispense; they must also set out the means to be used to ensure
that the provisions are met, and the penalties for contravention or
non-compliance. The purpose of the laws should be easy to understand
for all those affected by them, and ideally they should be simple and
clear. It is practical to establish the broad framework and mechanism
of control by comprehensive legislation, e.g. the Medicines Act in the
UK which empowers the minister to make statutory regulations on
details of implementation that do not need specific consideration
by the legislature. This arrangement facilitates the adaptation of
regulatory processes and practices to changing circumstances.

The alternative to laws and regulations is voluntary regulation.
This requires much less governmental time and manpower, but makes it
more difficult to ensure desired outcomes. It is therefore not
practicable where the individuals or companies affected are many
and heterogeneous, as are medical practitioners or pharmaceutical
manufacturers. Of course in the special case of a government monopoly
of medicine manufacture, the regulator and the regulated are different
arms of the same government apparatus, so that administrative control
can be complete, and legislation is hardly needed. Even so, external
audit is desirable, for one recognises that governmental services
function best when subject to independent scrutiny.

When general agreement cannot be achieved on the best system
of control, a compromise may be reached between voluntary and
legally enforceable regulation. For example, in the UK between 1964
and 1971 the scrutiny of new drugs by the Committee on Safety of
Drugs was not mandatory, but was performed by voluntary agreement
between the Association of the British Pharmaceutical Industry (ABPI)

and the Committee, which had been appointed by the Minister of
Health. The agreement bound members of the ABPI, but not companies
which did not belong to it. These were nevertheless under some
pressure to submit to the voluntary system, mainly because to do so
would help to protect them against charges of careless or negligent
drug testing and marketing that might arise if one of their products
turned out to cause harm. Participation in the voluntary scheme might
also have helped to improve the image of 'outsider' companies.

Another example from the UK is the control on the promotion of
medicines. Since 1958 the ABPI has had a Code of Practice governing
the promotion and advertising of products, which is binding on its
members (ABPI, 1979). When the Code was introduced its provisions
were relatively mild, but in successive revisions the rules have become
clearer and more stringent. More important, the procedure for implementing the code has become more effective. Initially the Code of
Practice Committee, which is responsible for deciding whether a
particular act by a company has contravened the Code, was entirely
made up of members from the industry, who found it difficult to be
tough with colleagues from offending companies. Complaints and
decisions about them were considered the private business of the
APBI. Although the Code probably did have a useful effect, it was not
seen in public to have any, and pressure from Parliament and successive
Health Ministers has recently led to a strengthening of the Code, and
to improvements in the composition and method of work of the Code
of Practice Committee. The Committee now has a barrister as an
independent chairman, and two of its members are doctors from
outside the pharmaceutical industry. Methods of bringing possible
infractions of the Code to the Committee's attention have been
improved; this is no longer left entirely to the initiative of outsiders.
The Committee still publishes very little about its decisions, and it has
no sanctions which it can impose on an offending company. But if the
Committee is not satisfied with the written answer to a complaint,
it asks the managing director of a company to attend in person and the
possible loss of face may be a deterrent. A voluntary system of this
kind has the great advantage that it is administered and paid for directly
by the industry, and costs the taxpayer very little (not nothing, because
some monitoring of manufacturers' promotional activity by civil
servants is still necessary, and the functioning of the system must
be reviewed regularly to ensure that it is adequately effective).

The informality of voluntary regulation also makes it much more
flexible. If a procedure is not working well, it is not too difficult to

change it. Regulations and laws that are ineffective cannot be changed so easily. It is therefore essential in the preparation of laws and regulations to consider all their implications and possible effects, and to consult well-informed representatives of all the groups who will be affected. In the case of licensing regulations it is most desirable to consult manufacturers, importers, exporters, prescribers, clinical pharmacologists, pharmacists, as well as representatives of those who consume medicines. Such consultations may require months of discussions and circulation of drafts, but deadlines may limit procrastination.

In principle voluntary regulation, like any self-discipline for the good of others, is far more reliable, effective and cheaper than external regulation. The task is to determine whether, in a given setting, there is sufficient harmony of implicit values, of an accepted priority of a community (national) interest, and a capacity for self-discipline. Many efforts at self-policing are exceedingly disappointing, whereas voluntary control of industrial conduct has a record ranging from grand to grotesque. It will be a wise public policy planner in the medicines sector who proceeds slowly to test voluntary systems, being sure to keep both carrot and stick close to hand. Insofar as some industrial participants may well owe their allegiance abroad (to some multinational headquarters) it is well to keep in mind that the local head of a company may be unable to comply if externally imposed business demands conflict with local voluntary agreements.

Balanced against the risks of voluntarism are the so well-known risks of government itself. Inherent in most bureaucracies, as studies show, are not just the advantages of specialisation, co-ordination, expertise and central authority, but great disadvantages as well. Parkinson's Law demonstrates these with sardonic humour — included are tendencies to unnecessary expansion, waste, concealment of activities, inefficiency, corruption and abuse of authority and failure to perform mandated services.

Once again the policy planner for medicines faces a real, not ideal, world in which it is as well to assume that there may be 'better' decisions but not 'best' ones, and that any system — *laissez-faire*, voluntary or self-policing, bureaucratic control or rule by edict and fiat — will exact its costs as well as provide (not always even that!) benefits. The modern manager will simply have to evaluate his own national setting and needs, the nature of the constituency, motives and capabilities of those acting in the system that provides and consumes medicines, and then using sense, opt for what appears to be workable and decent.

9.4.4 Ensuring Compliance with Regulations

The regulatory authority needs to know promptly about instances in which regulations are not being observed. For example, if an unlicensed medicine is being sold, the licensing authority must become aware of this: it therefore needs a mechanism for detecting such sales. When non-compliance has been detected, corrective action can be taken. The simplest is to inform the company or individual concerned that prompt compliance is required and to apply sanctions if it is not obtained. Prosecution is a last resort, and should rarely be needed. It is probably the most expensive method of enforcing regulations, in terms of money, civil service manpower, and of good will and co-operation from the regulated.

When a regulation is first introduced, and for quite a long time afterwards, the authority must devote much effort to detailed instruction and education of those who have to comply with it.

One example concerns the data to be submitted about a new product with an application for the product licence. In January 1980, at the fourth Symposium on Licensing Applications organised by the UK Department of Health, Dr G. Jones of the Medicines Division said that 'after 8 years of the Medicines Act, applications are still received for clinical trial certificates and product licences that are quite inadequate in terms of format and which have been compiled without paying due regard to the guidelines issued by the department'. He emphasised that 'some companies have a greal deal to learn' (*Scrip*, 1980).

A different and great educational problem is presented by unorthodox practitioners such as herbalists, homoeopaths and others who prescribe or administer medicines that are of unspecified composition and frequently unlicensed. In the UK a substantial proportion of the population use herbal, homoeopathic, or other unorthodox remedies. The Medicines Act applies to all these medicines, but at present there is no way of enforcing it. The practitioners who use them are so diverse and numerous, so inaccessible and so ignorant of the law and the reasons for it, that the only hope of improvement lies in prolonged and large-scale educational campaigns. In peasant or tribal societies it may be that most treatment is managed by family, community, or other non-medical healers. One need not assume that either mothers or folk-healers are utterly unsure in their choice of remedies, or that for minor diseases it matters much what they use as long as the patient is comforted and recovers in any event. But again education efforts are a prime requirement for any national medicines policy, not simply to help them avoid the waste of money or time on inert remedies (although granting these the normal, 40 per cent, placebo efficacy) but more importantly, to teach them to recognise those symptoms which require that competent healers be called in, so that medicines that *do* make a difference may be used.

One policy issue that has to be decided is how far to rely on trust and how far on detailed and costly supervision. How effective is trust when backed by severe penalties for non-compliance? The examples given show that in the face of ignorance trust is not an option. It is only possible when the regulated are clearly competent.

Compliance of companies with regulations is helped if a named individual with specified qualifications in the company is charged with the responsibility for it. For example, under the UK Medicines Act a company must make a pharmacist responsible for compliance with the regulations on quality control and good manufacturing practice. This not only facilitates inspection, but also makes it simpler to deal with the rare instances of fraud or falsification of data, when prosecution may be required. In a recent case in the USA, Biometric Testing Inc and three of its senior employees were convicted of conspiring to falsify reports to the FDA to show that certain drug products were harmless, when in fact the tests had not been performed (*Scrip*, 1979).

9.5 Regional and International Co-operation

Co-operation among countries both at the regional level as well as at an international level can greatly benefit all, by:

(1) Providing information on the status of the manufacturers in each country with regard to quality. This would minimise the risk of importation of poor-quality drugs, particularly by countries without facilities for quality control.

(2) Assisting in the setting-up of legal and administrative structures to implement national drug policies, particularly in developing countries.

(3) Training personnel for implementation of the various aspects of drugs policies as well as in the technical skills required for the production and quality control of pharmaceuticals.

(4) Developing an international monitoring system for adverse effects of drugs, and rapid evaluation and dissemination of

information on adverse effects, so that it will be possible to recognise such effects at the earliest possible moment and give early warning about them. The success of such a system depends primarily on the development of adverse-reaction monitoring centres at the national level.

(5) Developing consensus on high standards for the design of research – including data interpretation – so that one may someday assume uniform quality in the scientific work which constitutes drug screening and clinical trials. The public information derived from those trials, for all drugs rejected for reasons of toxicity or inefficacy, itself constitutes a body of scientific knowledge which should be accessible to national licensing authorities or to scientists asked to investigate post-registration (approval) reports on new adverse effects. Thus there is called for – we would propose under WHO auspices – an effective and well-financed information clearing-house for medicines. It need not itself be a data or journal library, but there should be a librarian capable of directing investigators, manufacturers, practitioners or national authorities to worldwide available data on the effects of any manufactured or commercially processed compound used in medical treatment.

(6) Establishment of Regional Co-operative Pharmaceutical Production and Technology Centre (COPPTECS), as proposed by Lall and UNCTAD and UNIDO (1978). This will greatly help countries with small markets and underdeveloped industrial resources. Such centres would function in the development of local pharmaceutical manufacture by co-ordinating production programmes so that production is economical. They would also act as channels for the transfer of technology and for providing information and guidance on questions covering importation of raw materials, production, training and marketing. Intergovernmental co-operation in checking on the quality of drugs manufactured in the region and maintenance of uniform quality control standards would also be of great value. Such regional centres could obtain assistance from international agencies such as UNCTAD, UNIDO and WHO which have the necessary technical information and expertise.

Regional and international co-operation on all these matters is still fragmentary, but increasing efforts are being made. Kay (1976) has reviewed the early development of these efforts concerning the control of quality of drugs in international commerce, the monitoring of adverse reactions, and drug information. Dukes (1979) describes the functioning of the Joint Benelux Services for the Registration of Medicines, which after a slow and shaky start is now firmly established and will from January 1981 handle all applications for licences in Belgium, Luxembourg and the Netherlands. He also outlines the steps which have been taken by the European Economic Community (EEC) to harmonise the approaches of its member states to various aspects of drug regulation. Up to the present their main value has been to encourage the member states to face the problems of regulatory discrepancies, to analyse the reasons for them, and to find common ground.

9.6 Concluding Remarks

In closing we offer the happy observation that the world seems reasonably well served by its drug providers, and that several different schemes for encouraging and controlling, nationally, medicines provision have evolved which appear to work well in their respective settings. There is a caution which we offer: it is that a reasonable interest in controlling greed or ignorance (both too evident in medicines manufacture or use) must not lead to control schemes which deter scientific discovery, drug invention itself.

The emphasis in this chapter on policy has focused, by accident of current need and definition, primarily on control and education to the exclusion of policies which encourage original development.

Certainly in those countries where there is neither basic science nor pharmaceutical industries with competition and capital assets allowing strong research and development departments, there has been no discovery of medicines. As worrying, in technologically advanced countries or others with competitive economies, there are pressures of inflation, sometimes anti-intellectualism, and such competition between general welfare needs and scientific support that basic science is losing out. Further, in the 'free market' (it is rarely that) industrial sector inflation has discouraged re-investment while controls and increased taxation may restrict the capital accumulation necessary for research. In this atmosphere patent theft, industrial espionage and unnecessary 'me too' drugs have become substitutes for real research as sources for new product development.

While there is not much that any drug policy administrator can do about some of these science-inhibiting factors of modern societies, we do make, as our final proposal, the recommendation that each participant in the complicated process of medicines provision define himself as a friend of research and discovery, industrial or academic, and do what he can to facilitate and support that basic work which we believe so important to improvements in health.

References

Arbon, J., Semler-Collery, J. and Simon, P. (1979). Pour un meilleur usage des médicaments. *La Revue de Médicine 24*, 11 June, 1232-4

Association of the British Pharmaceutical Industry (ABPI) (1979). Code of Practice. In Data Sheet Compendium 1979-80, London, ABPI

Australia: Commonwealth Department of Health (1979). Pharmaceutical benefits: schedule of benefits for medical practitioners. Canberra, August

Barker, C., Marzagão, C. and Segall, M. (1980). Economy in drug prescribing in Mozambique. *Tropical Doctor 10*, 42-5 (Published more fully in Portuguese in *Boletim: A Saude em Mozambique*, January and February 1978)

Deitch, R. (1980). Goodbye to the limited prescribing list. *Lancet, 1*, 1149

Dukes, M.N.G. (1979). The role of regional economic unions. In: *National Drug Policies (Public Health in Europe 12)*, Copenhagen, WHO Regional Office for Europe, 65-75

George, C.F. and Kingscombe, P.M. (1980). Can adverse drug reactions be prevented? *Adverse Drug Reactions Bulletin 80*

Gish, O. and Feller, L.L. (1979). Planning pharmaceuticals for primary health care: the supply and utilization of drugs in the Third World, *Monograph Series No 2*, Washington, American Public Health Association International Health Programs

Gross, F.H. and Inman, W.H.W. (eds.) (1977). *Drug Monitoring*, London, Academic Press

Inman, W.H.W. (ed.) (1980). *Monitoring for Drug Safety*, Lancaster, MTP Press

International Federation of Pharmaceutical Manufacturers Association (IFPMA) (1980). *Legal and Practical Requirements for the Registration of Drugs (Medicinal Products) for Human Use*, Zurich, IFPMA

Kay, D.A. (1976). The international regulation of pharmaceutical drugs. *Studies in Transnational Legal Policy 14*, Washington, The American Society for International Law

Knapp, D.A. and Palumbo, F.B. (1978). *Containing Costs in Third Party Drug Programs: Selected Bibliography and Abstracts*, Hamilton, Illinois, Drug Intelligence Publications

Medico-Pharmaceutical Forum (1978). Report of working party on the role of the pharmaceutical industry in postgraduate medical education. London, Medico-Pharmaceutical Forum

Scrip (1979). *446* (4), 12 December

Scrip (1980). *455* (3), 19 January

Symposium: Clinical Pharmacological Evaluation in Drug Control (1976). Copenhagen, WHO Regional Office for Europe

UNIDO (1978). *The Growth of the Pharmaceutical Industry in Developing Countries: Problems and Prospects*, New York, United Nations

United Kingdom (1968). Medicines Act

United Kingdom. Medicines Commission, Committee on Safety of Medicines, etc. Annual Reports

Wardell, W.M. (ed.) (1978). *Controlling the Use of Therapeutic Drugs, An International Comparison*, Washington, American Enterprise Institute for Public Policy Research
WHO (1977). The selection of essential drugs. WHO *Tech. Rep. Ser. 615*
—— (1979). Second Report. *Tech. Rep. Ser. 641*

INDEX